MOVING THE INTERNAL MATRIX

Revitalizing Fascia for Optimal Health and Well-Being

MOVING THE INTERNAL MATRIX

Revitalizing Fascia for Optimal Health and Well-Being

Libby Outlaw, LMBT

Founder of Fascial Conduction
Somatic Educator

Illustrated by Sue Sneddon
Foreword by Janice Geller

Mill City Press
Minneapolis, MN

Mill City Press, Inc.
322 First Avenue N, 5th floor
Minneapolis, MN 55401
612.455.2293
www.millcitypublishing.com

The information in this book is in no way intended to replace medical advice, diagnose or prescribe therapy to anyone. The purpose of this book is to provide information about the topic. The author and publisher are in no way liable or responsible for any injury, loss or damage due to the use of any of the information in this book. The author is not a medical authority and is not qualified to diagnose or prescribe any therapy. Please consult your physician concerning any medical conditions. The information in this book is the author's personal opinion from her own experience.

ISBN-13: 978-1-63505-080-6
LCCN: 2016910235

Cover Design by Jaime Willems
Cover Drawing by Sue Sneddon
Typeset by C. Tramell
Original Drawings of the Matrix by Sue Sneddon
Edited by Jeremy Hawkins
Photographs in *Self Practice* and *Hands-on Practice* by Cesar Carrasco

Printed in the United States of America

CONTENTS

Foreword vii

Introduction 1

PART I THE DYNAMICS OF FASCIA

Chapter 1. Anatomy of a Living Tissue 9

Chapter 2. Qualities of Fascia 32

Chapter 3. Density/Fluidity 35

Chapter 4. Slide and Glide 53

Chapter 5. Conductivity 71

Chapter 6. Layering/Compartmentalization 87

Chapter 7. Suspension/Buoyancy 102

Chapter 8. Coherence/Exchange 116

Chapter 9. Balanced Reciprocal Tension 130

Chapter 10. Liquid Crystalline Matrix 143

Chapter 11. The Body's Fractal Design 150

Chapter 12. Biotensegrity 160

Chapter 13. Fiber Connections 169

Chapter 14. Coherent Awareness, Consciousness and the Matrix 173

PART II APPLICATIONS

Chapter 15. Resources in the Body 182

Chapter 16. Stem Cells and Mesodermic Field Memory 184

Chapter 17. The Primitive Streak and Midline 190

Chapter 18. Heart Resonance and Coherence 195

Chapter 19. Inherent Health 199

Chapter 20. Self-Recognition 203

Chapter 21. Responsive Shifting Fulcrums 206

Chapter 22. Self-Practice 210

Chapter 23. Fascial Conduction: Hands-on practice 233

Chapter 24. Case Studies 260

Notes for Figures 267

Important Resources 271

Glossary 274

Index 280

About the Author 290

FOREWORD

BY JANICE GELLER, MA, LPC, LMBT, BC-DMT

With Moving the Internal Matrix: Revitalizing Fascia for Optimal Health and Well-being, Libby Outlaw leads us through an inner journey of somatic awakening. She asks us to awaken to the aliveness and connectivity that is possible within our whole body, when we bring awareness to the dynamic consciousness of our fascia.

Libby is a gifted somatic pioneer, who has created a new inspiring field of bodywork, which she has named Fascial Conduction. Libby proposes that we can find freedom in our own being, when we bring awareness to the internal vitalizing movement of our bodies, rather than be snared in the judging, planning, and obsessivte patterns of our mind. Libby explains in a compelling style, how limitations in the complexity of the internal facial matrix create discomfort, disease and pain, and gives us concrete ways to get out of, and stay out of pain. Libby links repetitive movement with pain and discomfort, and suggests that it is the diversity of movement that is a key to a healthy fascial matrix.

The book delves into the innovative bodywork of Fascial Conduction, providing fascinating concepts, accessible explorations and hands-on techniques, clarifying photographs, and real life case studies, to help us find ease in our own bodies, and find optimal health. A clear and fascinating discussion of the anatomy and physiology, the embryological development, and the density, conductivity and buoyancy of this unique tissue of fascia is explored. Libby is an organic farmer and gives illuminating parallels between the qualities of water, soil, and vegetation, and the qualities of fluid, density and wave like patterns within the body's fascial tissues. This innovative bodywork is applicable to everyone as a self-practice, as well as a hands-on technique for health professionals.

Libby and I met twenty years ago, and we have been friends and colleagues ever since. I have taken her Fascial Conduction classes, and received her powerful bodywork. As a Licensed Massage and Bodywork Therapist, and Body-Mind Centering Teacher and Practitioner, I know the deep benefits of her work, and use many concepts of the work with my clients. As a somatically oriented Licensed Professional Counselor, and Board Certified Dance Movement Therapist, I use the view of the fluidity of the internal matrix to inform and help my clients find comfort in their bodies, and develop acceptance of their thoughts and feelings.

Over the past ten years I have watched Libby develop Fascial Conduction. Libby is enthusiastic and thorough in her quest for knowledge, and is continually willing to integrate new information as the field grows and her perspective develops. Libby is able to understand complex scientific information and transform it into simple and accessible concepts, and create innovative movement explorations that everyone can utilize and understand. Libby's extensive study of the body, and understanding of her own fasical system, her extensive teaching, and her bodywork practice with clients for over thirty-five years, makes her an expert in this field. She leads the somatic profession, making great strides in expanding our awareness of the connectivity of the whole body, and the energetic field of awareness, which connects us with others in the world.

INTRODUCTION

Moving the Internal Matrix is an inquiry into the dynamic consciousness of fascia, which is the system of connective tissue within the body that connects, stabilizes, encloses and separates muscles and other human organs. Separate from the nervous system, fascia can provide us with its own unique information via its moving structures and coherent vibrations. However, very few people experience—let alone use—this information, which is vital to our shifting, adapting organism. Instead we spend most of our time focused inside the hierarchy of the mind: discerning, judging, planning and acting in life. This fast, frenetic pace of exchange in the world bypasses the vibrational level of being. This book is an invitation to change that.

Many times, when we think of *being* instead of *doing*, our minds interpret this as passive, no movement, inertia. Yet *being* (or what I will call *awareness*) is, in fact, a dynamic internal movement that can provide an expansive sensation of wellness, balance and interconnectedness. This internal movement is constant, yet it is always changing and adapting, fully experienced by all of our cells. It is our main source of knowing our place in the world. This internal movement of awareness, pure and simple, without commentary, soothes the soul and provides a counterpoint to anxiety, fear and emotional turmoil. When we shift our focus away from the daily routines and habitual patterns of stress and over-activity, and onto the full body, an awareness of life and our connections in the world, then we enter the space of the internal matrix.

This awareness, as experienced through the internal matrix of fascia, is the subtle underlying activity that supports and informs our movement through life. Our proprioceptors let us know where we are moving, and our muscles lever us through space, while our internal matrix readies us to move as one integrated form.

1

In life, movement is a constant. We move externally through space—limbs and torso gliding, twisting and turning to express our needs and take us where we want to go. We also move internally, with pulsations of heartbeat, breath and the constant shifting of our internal matrix of fascia.

When I investigate my own layers of movement, both externally and internally, I am constantly astounded by the variety of quality, direction, and the ebb and flow of movement within me. Our bodies hold an incredible capacity for expressing ourselves in movement, yet our minds often choose to limit this through habit and repetition. Do you know your limits, as well as your capacity for movement?

HOW THIS BOOK BEGAN

It is not an exaggeration to say that the roots of *Moving the Internal Matrix* are found in my youth, when I began my own exploration of life as movement through dance as a small child. Being left handed and somewhat knock-kneed, dance became a place where I could feel the inner messages of my own body without comparing it to others. I began to trust my body's ability to know how to move in complex ways with ease and glide.

As an adult, when I found my way into the bodywork profession, I shifted my focus to looking at the outside of the body and seeing the shaping and forming of a life in action. I was interested in the ways the neuromuscular system seems designed to contract or release in order to lever us through life, as well as its ability to hold and resist movement because of habitual patterns. One thing that continued to puzzle me was how those muscle fibers could "remember" their spatial relationship and engage in such complex, fast movement. As I moved into working more with the fascia and connective tissue, I saw how fascial tissue determines our capacity for diverse movement. I began to experience this fascial system as a another internal communication network, a network that seemed to be the missing piece around the movement complexity of our body.

After 40 years of listening, observing and touching the living body, I found a deep connection within this interconnected matrix in the body called fascia. Once I began engaging with this tissue and suggesting basic exercises to my clients, I began to see profound changes in my clients' quality of health, reduction of discomfort and limited range of motion, and overall engagement and vitality in life… and this has led me to look even deeper into this webbing of fascia.

THE INTERNAL MATRIX AND THE WHOLE ORGANISM

Our internal matrix of fascia is indeed a truly remarkable biological system, one we are just beginning to understand. Among its many amazing capacities, the internal matrix is able to shift and change very rapidly, providing our tissues both space and support for all manner of complex movements, both internal and external.

Jean-Claude Guimberteau, MD, a pioneering French surgeon and medical researcher, has shown, in a series of fascinating videos, how the rapidly shifting internal matrix functions at the microscopic level. Because of Guimberteau's research, as well as that of many other pioneers, we now understand that our internal fascial matrix is made up of millions of hollow threads of collagen, filled and interconnected with fluid, that continually shift and change their connecting points. These threads connect in icosahedron patterns that create a balanced tension between the points of connection and the tense strands in between. The shifting of these connection points is a continual dance of internal movement that resembles seaweed dancing in the ocean. With so many points of connection throughout our matrix, and with their ability to shift quickly and immediately, the matrix provides a means for both our large gliding movements through space, and our small, complex, fine motor movements.

In order for our internal matrix to be constantly aware of our whole organism, as well as be an information highway for our individual cells, it must provide a conductive pathway that is not only stable, but one that also shifts to include all new inputs from our internal and external environments. The matrix is able to perform these functions through the organized water that lines up between and within the microfibrils (see Chapter 1 for details). These microfibrils provide a surface of hydrogen molecules that organize the water between them. The electrons of the oxygen molecules within water are then pulled to the surface of the microfibril, giving the protons of the hydrogen molecules the ability to conduct through the matrix structure. Wave forms created from our internal functions pulsate through this conductive medium. When we experience these conductive pathways as a whole, we are experiencing our body's awareness of itself and of its surroundings.

As we will see, the internal matrix displays awesome versatility and dynamic balance. It is able to glide, spread and return to its resting configuration without pushing or pulling other tissues. Any time we move—reaching or pulling, turning or spiraling—the web responds so that our movement is fluid and connected.

This process is vitally important in all the functions of the human body. Almost all of our discomforts and diseases start with a limitation in the versatility and complexity of our internal matrix. For example, heartburn and indigestion start as a compression and lack of glide that spreads to the internal matrix surrounding the esophagus and stomach, reducing the ability of the digestive system to propel food down the gut tube. When working with a client that had GERD, I was able to reduce their symptoms by gliding the matrix under the rib cage and giving them internal movements to keep the matrix open and free of constriction. Frozen shoulder is another example; in this case, the internal matrix in the shoulder joint does not suspend the space between ligaments, bones and tendons to allow for a proper gliding motion, thus prohibiting arm movement in many directions. When I work with a frozen shoulder by gliding the matrix around the joint as well as at each of the rotator cuff attachments, I can gradually increase the complexity of the matrix and increase the range of motion in the shoulder.

The more complex the connections in the internal matrix, the greater the variety of movement and information exchange. Diversity of movement is one of the keys to a healthy matrix. The amazing complexity of the internal matrix found in the hands of a concert pianist demonstrates the potential of what our matrix is capable of.

My hope with *Moving the Internal Matrix* is to educate and engage you in this moving, shifting, conducting matrix, so that you can sense and feel its undulating movements, enhance its complexity, and settle into experiencing nonjudgmental awareness of your entire body.

REPAIRING OUR INTERNAL MATRIX

The internal matrix responds to and mirrors all of our activities and relationships in life. At first we organize movement functionally to be able to roll over, sit, stand and walk. As adults, our lifestyle tends to entail movements that are repeated throughout the day or on a regular basis. Sitting at the computer and typing away is a classic example; texting on a cell phone is another. Our habits in walking and sitting at work or in front of the TV solidify our internal matrix. We unconsciously fall into habitual patterns of movement that begin to limit the complexity and mutability of our matrix.

Pathological changes in our connective tissues occur as a result of these repetitive movement patterns. Specifically, such patterns can lead to a crosslinking of the collagen fibers that, in turn, causes them to bind together. As the matrix binds or rigidifies, the information flow to the cells diminishes, as well as the ability of the body to respond to changes in its environment. This underlying limitation begins to lessen the body's fluidity of movement through space, isolating pockets that are separate from the information flow. These areas of separation without vitality or adaptability are areas where degeneration and disease can manifest.

With our sedentary, repetitive, patterned lives we lose the sense of awareness, balance and vitality of the moving body. Hoping to find balance, we visit spas and health clubs that offer increased activity and orientation to the neuromuscular and cardiovascular systems, pumping our blood through our muscles, pulling on bones to create density, and building strength by increasing muscle cell size. These activities have helped usher in a whole new set of repetitive strains and injuries, limited range of motion, and fixed neuromuscular movement patterns. Weight training and treadmill-type movement are great for our heart and skeletal muscles, but through their repetitive, resistant movements, they reduce our capacity for diverse movement and adaptability in the world.

Further reducing such capacity is our lack of awareness of the internal movements that move and shape the fascia. Internal movement happens continuously in our daily life, without notice. As it is with external movement, so it is with internal. If the fascia is given only limited internal movement in which to respond, it will become limited. In order to truly open and use our movement potential, whether in relationship to range of motion, flexibility, stability, strength or endurance, the internal matrix must be enlivened to provide support and information to our integrated body.

I hope to change these unconscious habits and patterns, and to bring awareness and vitality to your moving experience by making the process of enlivening the matrix an integral part of your life and practice. To these ends, *Moving the Internal Matrix* will take you on a journey through your own body. I will guide you in exploring the internal movements of the matrix, identify qualities that you will want to enhance, and teach you to reach into a microscopic view of your collagen microfibrils.

Only through focus and attention on the internal matrix will you learn to experience a dynamic awareness of your body and participate in your interconnectedness within. By recognizing and experiencing your individual wave patterns resonating and vibrating through your matrix, you will begin to participate in shifting yourself from an unconscious, habitual, past-centered form to a diverse, multidimensional, interconnected being. As your awareness of the matrix grows, you will begin to influence its complexity and conductivity.

For those of you who are regular meditators, this work can enhance your capacity to shift from the mind's different states to a whole body awareness of the present moment. Meditation will support the expanded experience the internal matrix provides.

By connecting to your open, un-orchestrated qualities of movement, you will enhance your physical, mental, emotional and spiritual well-being. With an open readiness to respond to impulse, you will be at the doorstep of shedding past traumas and restrictions. You will become ever-present in our ever-changing world.

HOW TO USE THIS BOOK

Moving the Internal Matrix begins by exploring the anatomy and physiology of the fascia as a connective tissue (Chapter 1). Included in this exploration is the embryology that forms the fascia in the developing embryo. As you learn about the workings of the matrix, you will be guided to a deeper understanding via language, metaphor, guided explorations and guided meditations. With this experiential context for exploring the fascia, you will achieve both visual and kinesthetic understanding of the internal matrix and its balance between compression and suspension.

Next you will be led to directly experience the qualities of the fascia that shape and form how we move, explore, digest and exchange (Chapters 2-14). Separate chapters will illuminate the qualities of density, slide and glide, conductivity, coherence, suspension and balanced reciprocal tension. (Definitions for these terms can be found in the Glossary.) I will guide you in exploring each quality from within your body, within your movement, and within your hands.

With regular practice of the Explorations found in these chapters, you will begin to notice and experience the various qualities of fascia. Your body will feel more balanced and integrated, your step lighter, and your system more ready to respond to the external stimuli in our world. You will experience more of your internal movement/internal web, and you will begin to exert a conscious influence upon it. The sensations of your body will change as well. Where you have noticed pain or discomfort, pressure or strain, a new sense of freedom and integration will arise. Your movements will begin to feel more fluid and increasingly effortless.

Finally, *Moving the Internal Matrix* will provide specific applications to build a felt sense and direct experience of your internal matrix (Chapters 15-22). By creating a felt sense of your matrix, you will awaken your capacity to experience a clear, open state of awareness without being "censored" by your mind. Such a state of awareness is the medium wherein pure consciousness resides. This felt sense of consciousness allows us to disengage from our judging and dissecting minds and to enter into a place of calm, peaceful tranquility.

When you practice being in awareness and letting consciousness arise, your system will recalibrate to the present moment and will let go of repetitive physical and emotional reactions to life. You will experience life with greater ease, flow and equanimity. Your body will be ready to respond and adapt to the external and internal forces of life in a more open, present and resilient way.

I hope that you will enjoy exploring your internal information highway, the internal matrix of fascia.

Note for bodyworkers and other hands-on professionals: A collection of hands-on techniques and case studies can be found at the end of this book (Chapters 23-24).

CHAPTER 1
ANATOMY OF A LIVING TISSUE

To understand the anatomy of the fascia—from its webbing within the body to its microscopic microfibril orientation—I invite you to engage your imagination in a new way: Think of your body's tissues as alive, dynamic and ever-moving. If you focus on the internal sensations of your body, under the skin and between the organs, you can feel or at least imagine the ebb and flow movements. When you learn to listen to your matrix, you will actually be listening to your own recorded history, your past responses and relationships to your internal and external environments, all of which have been recorded in your body.

Life's movement over time is a series of shifting patterns in the internal matrix of relationship, and the body serves as the medium that moves us through this timeline. The body is shaped and informed by interactions with the internal and external environment. These interactions determine the container for our functioning fluids and tissue systems, and this container, a reflection or manifestation of the activities of life, is the three-dimensional bioelectric matrix of the fascia, a type of mesodermic connective tissue. Fascia is a moving, vibrationally responsive tissue that shifts and changes with every input, function and movement of our body. Fascia pulsates our own signature wave pattern continually, without pause.

You are a unique individual, shaped and informed by your history, relationships and activities. Your history is integrated in the overall wave pattern that pulsates through your fascial webbing. I call this the *signature wave* of an individual. You can sense this signature wave when a person enters the room or you make contact with them. Although we may not be conscious of the vibration of that person, we respond by moving toward them, being wary or withdrawing from them, because of our response to their signature wave.

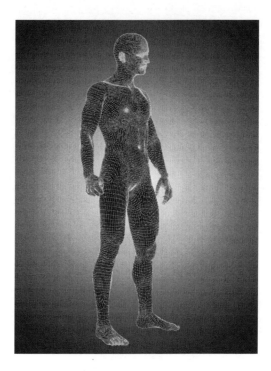

Fig. 1 Fascial Web

The internal matrix of fascia is a fascinating tissue with many layers, qualities and metaphors that reflects our history, our movement, and how we engage with our environment. The different qualities of fascia are consistent, from the tiniest quantum levels and microscopic ionic elements, to the visible matrix structure. All of these qualities determine the vitality, versatility and diversity of movement in our fascial matrix. So let's look at this living, moving matrix of fascia in detail, from structural, functional, embryological and field perspectives.

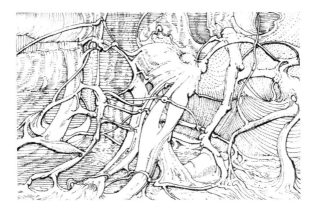

Fig. 2 Drawing of Fascial Matrix

WHAT IS FASCIA?

Fascia is a type of connective tissue that creates an interconnected matrix, or webbing, throughout the human body.

The matrix can be differentiated into layers, all of which are interconnected. On the surface, just beneath the skin, is a superficial double layer of fascia that creates the contours of the body and a pocket for surface nerves and vessels to reach the outer boundaries of our bodies.

The next layer forms the pockets for muscles, tendons and ligaments. This so-called *myofascia* surrounds our muscular and skeletal systems, including muscle fibers, muscle bundles, muscle groups, tendons and ligaments. This fascia also connects to the periosteum surrounding our bones.

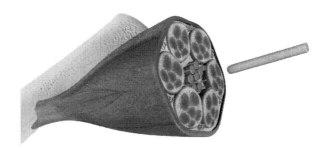

Fig. 3 Myofascial Layers

The next layer is known as the *visceral fascia*, which creates space for the organs, separating and individuating them. The visceral fascia gives organs the ability to act independently yet remain in communication with the whole organism.

Finally, the deepest layer of fascia—which forms from both mesoderm and ectoderm stem cells—surrounds the spinal cord and brain. This deep layer is called the *dura mater* or *dural tube*. When the dural tube enters the cranium it becomes the membranes in the brain known as *falx celebri, falx cerebelli,* and *tentorium cerebelli*). Cerebral spinal fluid moves between the cranium and sacrum within this deep layer of fascia.

These different fascial layers separate living tissue systems so that they can function independently, while the fascial matrix acts as an information highway between them. These layers generally organize longitudinally as a response to gravity, helping to differentiate and protect the enveloped structures. All of the layers create space and relationship from skin to bone, while also allowing the other tissue structures to move and glide independently. Thus the fascia is an integrated and interconnected matrix, touching all tissue surfaces, conducting and exchanging information between them.

There are also horizontal webbings of fascia that help to stabilize and anchor the fascia system, giving it more strength, resistance, and the ability to move within the vertical force of gravity. These webbings are also known as *horizontal diaphragms*, of which there are three main types: (1) the pelvic diaphragm in the pelvic bowl of the lower abdomen; (2) the respiratory diaphragm at the solar plexus; and (3) the shoulder diaphragm, where the torso and neck meet. There are other areas of horizontal webbing at the joints, all helping to create stability to an ever-moving system. This horizontal webbing is organized multi-directionally, giving diverse stability and strength to the system.

"Support in a moving structure arises from the organization and arrangement of the connective tissues."

–From The Endless Web: Fascial Anatomy and Physical Reality*,* **R. Schultz** *&* **R. Feitis, North Atlantic Books, pg. 32.**

HOW TO USE THE EXPLORATIONS IN THIS BOOK

The Explorations in this book are invitations to turn your mind away from your busy life and focus on the internal sensations in your body. By letting your mind engage in observing, listening to, and connecting with the different internal movements of your body, you will begin to inform—and be informed by—your body's experience of life. It will be important to suspend your preconceived notions and "expertise" and let your body be your guide.

Think of these Explorations as the first step in a long, meditative, creative process. If, for example, you cannot "find" the internal spaces discussed in a certain Exploration, you could search for an image online or create your own image for what your are exploring. Accuracy is irrelevant. Sensation differentiation is paramount.

Start by reading each Exploration thoroughly so you know what it is you are to focus on. Spend some time shifting your awareness from your normal, cause-and-effect, conscious thought patterns to letting your mind focus on the aspect of your body the Exploration is guiding you through. Let your mind describe the internal sensations you are experiencing and differentiate between them. Words such as warm, cold, pulsating, jumping, dense, hard, soft, slick or sticky are useful descriptions of the sensations you might have.

Go through the Exploration slowly, giving time to notice sensations and giving time for the body to guide and express its experience. Repeat to gain new levels of experience.

Allow the body to move on its own without commentary, judgment or direction from the mind. Continue to shift from thinking about your body to a meditative awareness of the experience.

Finish each Exploration in stillness and observing. Then get up and move to feel how your body has shifted. Remember your experience and apply it to your daily activity.

Enjoy exploring your internal matrix!

EXPLORATION 1: SHIFTING FROM MUSCLE MOVEMENT TO FASCIAL MOVEMENT

(See Warm up in Self Practice, pg. 213 for more description and illustrations)

We will begin by shifting focus from the movement of the neuromuscular system to the fascial system.

To start, use your muscles to move through space. From a standing position, begin by flexing and extending your arm at the elbow. Feel the contracting and releasing of the biceps as you bring your forearm closer to your upper arm. As you bend and straighten the arm, feel the muscles shortening and lengthening in order to move your arm through space.

Now begin to mindfully move your whole body across the room. Feel the neurological integration of movement as your legs and arms move in a contralateral pattern, moving forward and back to create walking. Notice your joints as the fulcrums, the long bones as the levers. Notice how as one muscle contracts, others must release to allow for movement.

Next, shift from simply moving forward to side-to-side, then backwards. Notice how smoothly your muscles coordinate their actions. Shift to stretching, reaching, pushing and pulling, feeling the strength and coordination in the neuromuscular system.

Now come back to your standing position. Feel how the neuromuscular system has warmed up your body, pumping the blood and lymph, warming the fascia as well.

Now let's concentrate on movement in the fascial system. From the standing position, use one hand to hold the other wrist, gently moving (gliding) the arm away from the wrist and toward the shoulder until you feel tautness (but not a muscular stretch). Slowly let go of your wrist and feel the spring-like quality of the fascial tissue as it comes back to its original position. This requires some practice, so don't be alarmed if you don't feel it right away.

(Continues on next page.)

Now gently rotate (glide) the arm, spiraling the fascia around the bones. Hold onto the wrist while rotating within the space of the arm. While holding the wrist, glide the fascia up the arm and let that extend through the shoulder, across the upper back, and down the other arm. Repeat with your other arm. These movements are internal and small. You have to continue to let go of moving all of the tissues in the arm or pushing through the tissues so your matrix can start to glide between the other tissues.

Now raise one arm up to the side of your head, pulling gently from the fingertips at a diagonal upward, feeling the tautness move down the arm, across the torso and down the opposite leg. You may need to adjust your pull from the fingertips to continue the sensation of tautness through to the opposite leg. Glide back and forth, keeping the movement within the diagonal space. Keep letting go of moving the whole arm and let the webbing glide within the arm. Imagine your webbing to be a sleeve moving over the internal surfaces of the body.

Repeat on the other side. Notice the difference between moving through space and within space, between levering and gliding.

MICROFIBRIL/ORGANIZED WATER MATRIX

As we've discussed, the different structures within the fascia allow it to be strong and stable, as well as mutable and adaptable to inputs from internal and external environments. These fascial structures arrange themselves into a conductive pathway where the vibrations and internal movements of the body entangle to create a *signature wave pattern* for each living being. This signature wave pattern vibrates to every cell of the body, reflecting the integrated wholeness of the organism in each moment, as well as immediately reflecting the shifts and changes in our individual and global biosphere.

The internal structure of fascia consists of three parts: (1) ground substance, (2) various cells and molecules, and (3) collagen fibers. The *ground substance* is a semi-fluid, somewhat gelatinous medium that provides a slickness for the tissues it surrounds to slide and glide between. It also allows for the movement of nutrients and toxins between the cells and the blood. The viscosity of the ground substance varies with temperature, pressure and structural needs, and the density of the ground substance is a factor in the overall fluidity, adaptability and mutability of the fascial matrix.

The second internal structure in the fascia is the cells and molecules within the fascia. This includes a complex array of nutrients, toxins, hormones, blood components and nerve cells, including proprioceptor, pain and autonomic sympathetic motor fibers. One of the most important cells in the fascia is the *fibroblast*. Along with many other functions, fibroblasts form the tropocollagen molecules (triad formations with hollow centers) which become the collagen fibers in the matrix.

FIBROBLAST

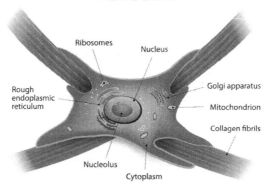

Fig. 4 Fibroblast

The final part of the fascial structure is the collagen matrix of fibers formed from the tropocollagen molecular structures created by the fibroblasts. These individual tropocollagen structures connect and stack together to form microfibrils. As they stack together, they rotate to form a spiraled structure with a hollow center and an internal and external surface of hydrogen atoms. The microfibrils continue this spiraling and come together to form collagen fibers, which then connect at multiple points to form the webbing of fascia.

This formative dance of collagen fibers continues throughout our lives as fibers are replaced, repaired and created. They spiral together, connect and disconnect, and respond to the movements of life. On the microfibril level a microscopic dance of conductivity is formed and continues throughout our lives.

The microfibrils create the structure for the dynamic, conductive pathway of the matrix. These spirals are designed so that the hydrogen atoms in their molecular structure line up on the inside and outside of their form. This invites a unique relationship to form with the water molecules around them. Water fills the spaces inside and outside of the microfibrils, organizing their H_2O molecules around the hydrogen surfaces. In these confined spaces, water is organized into a coherent, structured domain. This coherence allows the protons of the hydrogen atoms to dislocate and conduct through the organized water, "jumping" in and out of the chain. This is known as the *proton pump*, which acts like a semiconductor, moving energy faster than electricity. This highly conductive, coherent domain vibrates at the signature wave of the organism.

Through the work of Mae-Wan Ho and other physicists and biologists, we have a greater understanding of this amazing living structure and how it creates its own information highway for the body.

Mae-Wan Ho, Ph.D.: "The collagen-rich liquid crystalline mesophases in the connective tissues, with their associated structured water, therefore, constitutes a semi-conducting, highly responsive network that extends through the organism. This network is directly linked to the intracellular matrices of individual cells via proteins, as well as water channels that go through the cell membrane. The connective tissues and intracellular matrices, together, form a global tensegrity system as well as an excitable electrical continuum for rapid intercommunication throughout the body."

–From *The Rainbow and the Worm: The Physics of Organisms*, World Scientific, pg. 232.

This matrix of microfibrils surrounded by organized water creates an internal conductive pathway for wave patterns, protons and photons. These layers of collagen strands can bind and release water molecules at the elemental level, which gives the matrix the ability to change shape and relationship, adapting to the pressure and tension in the living body. The fascial matrix is strong but flexible, because of its *biotensegrity pattern* (similar to the multi-sided, vacuole-like structures as seen in Buckminster Fuller's architectural work [See Chapters 10, 11 and 12].

At every moment, millions of microfibril connections are shifting and re-connecting, conducting wave pattern and functional changes throughout the body. This relationship between the microfibrils and the H_2O molecules is constantly changing in response to the internal and external changes in the environment. Water molecules hold microfibrils together, slide between the fibrils, and break free to allow for different connections to form. The conductive wave in the internal spaces of the microfibrils, along with the connecting and disconnecting between them, creates the dynamic moving structure of the fascia. The level of movement inside and outside the matrix varies; the more diverse and complex the movement, the more vibrant and enlivened the body becomes as a whole. In this book, our primary focus will be on the conductive capacity of this microfibril/organized water matrix.

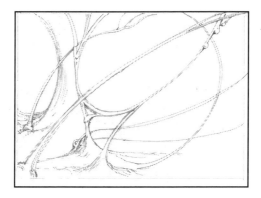

Fig. 5 Drawing of Internal Matrix

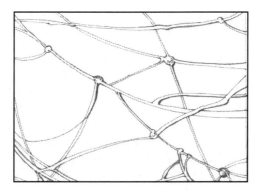

Fig. 6 Microfibrils in the Matrix

EXPLORATION 2: FINDING YOUR FASCIAL MATRIX

Find a comfortable place to lie down on the floor and settle into your body. Focus your awareness inside your body. Imagine a webbing throughout your body, from under the skin around your organs and muscles and deep around your bones and spinal cord. Imagine them interconnected so that with each impulse of movement the matrix responds.

Initiate a small gentle movement from your torso and follow that movement through the webbing. Continue to let go of trying to move your body and let it move itself. Try to feel, at a very subtle level, the movement of the fascial matrix under your skin as you glide the superficial sleeve of fascia. Feel the sleeve move around other tissues. This requires a blend of sensitivity, intuition and imagination.

Imagine you can move inside your own body, and that you can literally see the matrix of fibers. Notice the webbing of collagen fibers around the solid forms, like a mesh bag that has compartments filled with solid structures. Imagine you can enter this tissue microscopically and swim through the ground substance. Notice the viscosity of the fluid. Notice the different cells suspended in the fluid. Find the fibroblast, nutrient, toxin, hormone, blood or nerve cell. Enter with your imagination into the micro-level of the collagen strands and notice the matrix of micro-fibril strands surrounded by water. Feel the movement within this like seaweed floating in the water.

Imagine swimming in the waters between the microfibrils, like swimming in a mass of seaweed in the ocean. Go deeper into the body and notice the organization of the matrix as it surrounds the solid structures of organs, muscles and bones you are circling. Finally, bring your awareness back from the microscopic level of water and microfibrils to the webbing under the skin, then to the sensations of your whole body. Gently open your eyes and notice how your felt sense of the body has changed.

WHAT IS THE FUNCTION OF FASCIA?

- Connect all tissues of the body

- Differentiate and protect structures

- Create space for tissue to inhabit and maintain function

- Create a medium for metabolic, electromagnetic and stimulus exchange

- Create resonant and conductive pathways for heartbeat, breath, cranial wave and other wave patterns

- Ability to adapt and change matrix to shifting external and internal forces

- Create a dynamic integrated webbing that responds to energetic, bioelectric and piezoelectric inputs

- Maintain a balanced reciprocal tension between suspension and coherence within tissues

---

"Ideally, movement from a gesture travels through the arm or leg or head toward the spine. Movement transmits as a wave down the spine as well as across the spine and into the other side of the body. Thus, when the arm moves, that movement should continue wavelike through the neck and into the head."

–From *The Endless Web: Fascial Anatomy and Physical Reality*, R. Schultz & R. Feitis, North Atlantic Books, pg. 29.

EXPLORATION 3: MOVING THE FUNCTIONAL MATRIX

(See Gliding the fascia in Self Practice, pg. 214 for more description and illustrations)

Lying supine, let your body relax into the floor; feel the support from the floor. Feel the outline of your body. Focus on the inside of the skin where the fascial sleeve surrounds, shapes and encapsulates the internal systems.

Gently glide the superficial fascia by subtly pulling up through the legs, torso, head and arms. Let the glide move past the solid structures underneath, spreading and drawing upward to the head. Feel how the fascia glides over the deeper layers, maintaining the internal space. This is a small surface movement. You can flex the foot to aid in the movement, and you can stretch your neck and head slightly to enhance the glide.

Glide back down to the feet, gently pulling down from the leg and the back of your heel. Again, feel how the matrix shifts and moves to the internal movement, sliding by the solid structures beneath it.

Now bring your awareness to the middle layers of fascia surrounding the organs, muscles or bones. Glide gently by pulling the right hip downward, letting the webbing around the liver under the right rib cage move and spread around the solid organ. Notice how the webbing shifts and moves. See how far away from the hip you can sense the matrix. Use small gliding internal movements. Let your matrix move you.

Now simply let go and let your body relax and settle. Focus on your matrix and let it initiate slow gliding movements within the space of your body in any direction. You can bring a gentle stretch to an area to begin the movement. Stay relaxed and let the matrix move itself. When you feel your muscles engaging, pause and relax, letting the internal matrix initiate a new movement.

Notice how the matrix suspends and reorganizes, pulls together and releases as it moves. Notice how the whole body moves as one matrix, each impulse rippling through it. When your body comes to stillness notice how your body sensations have changed as well as your awareness of your internal body. Notice the enlivening of the body and the pulsations and wavelike patterns that move through the functional matrix.

WHAT IS THE FUNCTION OF THE MICROFIBRIL/ORGANIZED WATER MATRIX?

- To create a conductive matrix that is interconnected at the micro-level

- To conduct the signature wave pattern of the body

- To respond to the movements within the body

- To form and unform in order to maintain the balanced reciprocal tension of suspension and coherence

- To create a crystalline memory so the matrix can return to its place of neutral (neutral is the balance between the matrix and the force of gravity)

HOW DOES FASCIA DEVELOP IN THE EMBRYO?

The way our bodies develop from the fertilized egg to the embryo and fetus is an amazing journey fueled by tensions and pressures that guide cellular development and ultimately shape and construct tissues. Embryonic cells develop into tissues and organs growing from the three types of stem cells: ectoderm, mesoderm and endoderm. The fascia grows from the mesoderm, which develops between the ectoderm and endoderm once the embryo has attached to the uterus.

The mesoderm is formed on day 15 of development, when the bilaminal disc formed by the ectoderm and endoderm receives the first impulse of life from the primitive streak. This impulse is a wave of motion that gathers nutrients as it passes between the ectoderm and endoderm, forming the mesoderm. The primitive streak then sets up orientation for cells to form the left and right sides of the body as the mesodermic stems cells create pockets and containers for the other tissues of the body. This impulse is the first wave motion of life that continues in the internal matrix throughout our life.

All connective tissues are created from the mesodermic layer of the embryo. As mentioned previously, fascia is a type of connective tissue that arises from the first pulsation of life before becoming the conduit for the fluids and wave motions in the body. The deepest layer of fascia, including the dural tube and membranes of the head, are created through the ectoderm and mesoderm.

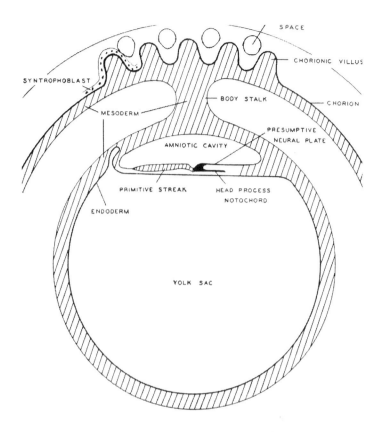

Fig. 7 Primitive Streak in embryo

"The 'organ' that transmits movement in the body, that makes a structural whole, is the mesodermic tissues."

–**From** *The Endless Web: Fascial Anatomy and Physical Reality*, **R. Schultz & R. Feitis, North Atlantic Books, pg. 27.**

WHAT IS CONNECTIVE TISSUE?

All connective tissue is derived from the mesoderm, orienting and developing out of the midline. All connective tissues have the same three structures:

ground substance, cells and collagen fibers. Connective tissues vary the relationship of these three structures in order to meet their individual functional needs.

Connective tissue includes bone, muscle, fascia, tendon, ligament, intervertebral discs, heart muscle, respiratory diaphragm, lymph, blood and sheaths around nerves. Ligaments and tendons have more collagen fibers to create support and strength, while blood has more ground substance for transporting nutrients throughout the body. Although they are different tissues with different functions, collagen fibers can connect between the different connective tissues. This relationship is clearly seen between the fascia and muscles, muscles and tendons, tendons and bones. This gives the movement fibers a communication network that is separate but engaged with the sensory motor nervous system. This interwoven webbing of fibers creates a continual matrix of relationship and interconnected mesodermic field.

ENERGY, FIELD, RESONANCE AND CONDUCTION

In exploring the fascia, it is important to understand the unseen forces that ripple and pulsate within its crystalline matrix. Energy fields that vibrate within the fascial matrix begin with the primitive streak, binding the matrix to the mesodermic stem cell field, the connective tissue field and the coherent vibratory field.

By looking at the morphogenetic field (the field of energy that develops and maps itself within the organism through time) we begin with the mesodermic field that the matrix develops out of, and continue through the resonant field that vibrates through its conductive medium. From this energetic level, we can understand the unique importance of the fascial matrix and its connection to the integrity and vitality of the body.

*res·o·*nance

- **the quality of a sound that stays loud, clear and deep for a long time**

- **a quality that makes something personally meaningful or important to someone**

- **a sound or vibration produced in one object that is caused by the sound or vibration produced in another from online *Merriam Webster Dictionary***

WHAT IS AN ENERGY FIELD?

A field can be defined as *energy organized around a function, intention or fulcrum*. The field, in turn, manifests as a semipermeable, invisible, non-physical membrane, attracting toward it all that enhances its function and repelling all that diminishes it.

There are many different types of energy fields. Some carry electrical charge, some carry memory, and some are created by the rhythms of life. These electrically charged fields create a conductive container for information and wave motion to move from field to field. *Fascial function* is determined collectively by the morphogenetic, mesodermic, bioelectric and conductive fields. As you explore and touch fascia using the Explorations in this book, you will enter experientially into these various fields of bio-energetic relationship.

Conductive field

The *conductive field* is a field that can take an impulse and vibrate it through a structure or medium. The microfibrils of the fascial system create the framework for the conductive field by loosely binding H_2O. This organizes water into a conductive medium, providing channels for impulse and vibration to move through. These channels conduct all the wave motions and vibrations of the body to every cell.

Bioelectric field

The *bioelectric field* is a unified field of relationship. This field is charged with + and - ions that create attracting and repulsing forces that, when aligned in certain ways, allow for continual pulsation through its structure.

In the human body, the microfibril/organized water matrix provides a bioelectric field. This field continually pulsates the signature wave of the organism, connecting the body to the electric and magnetic fields inside and out.

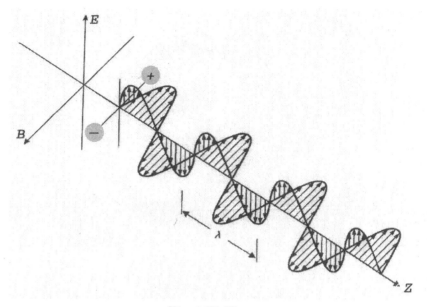

Fig. 8 EMF wave

Mesodermic field

The *mesodermic field* is the embryological resonance found in all mesodermic tissue. It invokes the qualities of the primitive streak (or first wave of life), the midline of the body, and the connection of the three types of stem cells. It is a resource for the connective tissue to maintain its mutability and adaptability. These qualities of energy are embedded in the internal matrix of fascia. They are the inherent qualities that the internal matrix continues to create throughout its life.

Morphogenetic field

The *morphogenetic field* is the resonance of a system that continues through time, creating an energetic memory expression. The morphogenetic field of memory that resonates in the fascial matrix supports the microfibrils' ability to complexify and modify in response to pressure, tension and movement.

Fascial field

All of these fields interconnect in the *fascial field*, creating a continual flow of information and resonance in the body.

The fascial field is organized around several key components:

- The movement of waves and impulses through the structure

- The suspension and coherence in the body

- A unified bioelectric matrix

- The body's responses to movement and pressure

- The informing of all cells continually

- The flow in and out of the midline

- The individual's signature wave

- The vibrational information network of the body

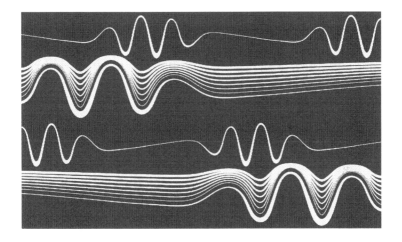

Fig. 9 Wave Patterns

EXPLORATION 4: FEELING THE CONDUCTIVE FIELD

Begin by rubbing your hands together, charging the static electricity through the piezo effect. With your palms facing each other a foot apart, bring them slowly together until you feel the push and pull of the energy between them. If you have magnets, bring them together slowly feeling the conductive pull between them.

Now put your hands on your chest. Feel the conductive flow, the drawing together and apart of the energy between your hands and your chest. Follow that flow into the body and notice when it shifts and moves. Glide the internal matrix by gently pulling down from the mid-back to accentuate the conductive flow. Follow the flow of energy between your hands and your chest. Let your imagination and felt sense discover the subtle wave motion in the field.

Put your hands on the center of your abdomen. Notice the conductive flow between your hands and your abdomen. Notice the movement, rhythm and direction of the energy in the abdomen. Let that conductive flow move your internal matrix as you follow the rippling pulsation.

Initiate small pulsations from any part of the internal matrix. Notice how the pulsation ripples through the conductive medium of the fascia. Feel the ripples move through the microfibril pathways. It you are not sensing the subtle pulsations, imagine the complex wave patterns flowing through the matrix. Imagine them as waves in the ocean, flowing through the matrix.

With your hands at your sides, let the internal matrix begin to move and feel the conductive flow within it. Let that flow move out to the surface of your body and feel its outer flow creating the energy field around you. Let it flow back to your midline.

Come to stillness and notice the conductive field. Notice the different sensations in your body.

RESONANCE

In the body, our so-called *resonance* is a vibration or frequency that changes continually through internal and external inputs. That vibration is conducted through cell microtubules and through the microfibril/organized water matrix of the fascia. All the different layers of internal rhythmic wave motion (breath, heartbeat, Cranial rhythm, mid and long tide) create an integrated wave motion that joins with the vibrational inputs of the functioning tissues. These together create the resonance or signature wave of the body, vibrating continually through the fractal layers of the microfibril/organized water matrix. This resonance is a strong, deep and clear vibration found in all living things.

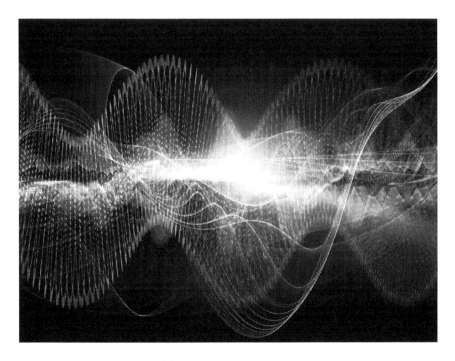

Fig. 10 Wave patterns

EXPLORATION 5: FIELDS OF RESONANCE AND LAYERS OF WAVE IN THE BODY

Find a comfortable position, either sitting or lying down, then settle and relax into the space you inhabit. Bring your awareness to your internal matrix and imagine you can feel, see or hear the wave motion throughout its layers. Move your imagination past the structure as it dissolves into it wave motion.

Focus on your heartbeat. Place your hand on an artery or near your heart where you can feel your heart beating. Notice that its rhythm is quick and steady: 60 to 80 beats a minute. Imagine the arterial flow of blood out to the extremities, and the venous flow pulsing back to the heart. Imagine you can separate its wave motion from the complex wave flow in your matrix. Then let your concentration dissolve back into your complex wave motion.

Now focus on the breath. Feel how it moves and ripples through your whole body as you inhale and exhale. The rhythm is slower and longer, six to 10 breaths a minute.

Focus on the cranial wave that flows from the sacrum up the dural tube into the membranes of the brain and back. Feel how it expands and contracts, rotating around your midline at about eight to 14 cycles per minute.

Next, focus on the midline tide as it slowly moves in and out of the midline at two to three cycles per minute. Imagine the slow wave motion that ebbs and flows from your midline, like ocean waters coming to the shoreline.

Focus on the long tide as it moves very slowly up the body from the toes up the legs and torso out the head into the universal flow around you, taking 50 seconds to a minute to flow through your matrix.

From this deepest, slowest rhythm, move back through each faster rhythm until you are back to the heartbeat.

Feel these different rhythms meet each other in the matrix and begin to wave together. Feel your singular wave pattern resonating in your micro-fibril/organized water matrix.

Finally, return to total stillness, simply watching the ebb and flow of your breath. Notice the changes in your internal sensations and your new awareness of your signature wave.

THE BRIDGE BETWEEN STRUCTURE AND FIELD

The structure and field of fascia create a living tissue system that supports, responds and conducts the processes of the living organism. They interface and mirror each other throughout the life of the organism. Through the embryological stage, they work to create the functioning organism and its ability to live and move in the environment surrounding it.

In the lifetime of the organism, the *structure* relates to the needs of the moment, while the *field* is the resource and potency of the body. The conductive pathways of the microfibrils that are always shifting and changing create the bridge between structure and field.

All of the different formations of collagen fibers that come from fibroblasts are determined by the functional need of the connective tissues they support. This varies not only in the embryological stage, but also during the lifetime of expression and patterning for the organism. The structure, size and type of collagen fibers change whenever the pressure and tension in the system demand it. This mutability in the fiber structure diminishes as we age and habitual patterns become more rigid.

The ability of microfibrils to connect and disconnect, while simultaneously maintaining a conductive and supportive medium, plays a crucial role in the potency, vitality and adaptability of our bodies. This bioelectric matrix of microfibrils and organized water provides a dynamic aliveness to our organism. It creates a bridge between the collagen fiber structure and the field of relationship that gives the body the ability to be conscious and aware of the relationship between its manifest structure and its energetic wave pattern. Moreover, the organism uses this relationship between structure and field to connect to the larger biosphere of the Earth. Though this relationship can be diminished by the pressures and repetitive patterns of life, it can also be enlivened by revitalizing the microfibril/organized water matrix.

By moving the internal matrix and experiencing its dynamic structure and energetic field, we can enter into a relationship with consciousness and shift our perceptions, proprioception and conscious expression in life. This allows us to act and choose in life outside of the habitual patterning found in our nervous system, giving us the ability to live in the present moment.

CHAPTER 2
QUALITIES OF FASCIA

Now that you have a basic understanding of the dynamic field and structure of the fascial matrix, we can use this foundation to explore the fascia's different qualities, in particular those qualities that can engender a healthy, enlivened body. These qualities vary in relationship to the functional needs of the surrounding tissues, as well as the body's degree of health and vitality.

Your daily habits of posture and movement can enhance or inhibit the enlivened capacity of the fascial matrix, and this in turn can determine the health and well-being of your entire body. When you work all day at a computer or stand all day as a teacher, the fascia binds to hold your positions throughout the day. But when you vary your movement and incorporate movements that are not in the traditional, forward moving realm of everyday life, the matrix is more diverse and adaptable, and thus healthy.

When evaluating a person's overall health at the tissue level, we look at three fundamental dimensions: (1) potency, (2) vitality and (3) adaptability. These dimensions of whole body health are the underlying factors that give us the capacity to meet challenges and deal with the changes in our lives.

Potency might also be called resilience, because it allows us to continue when we are stressed, fatigued or energy deprived. This can be crucial when we are faced with working overtime, finishing a project or navigating a crisis. Potency is the reserve that we can harness when our normal energy output is depleted.

Vitality allows us to respond appropriately to stimuli in our world. This gives us the ability to stay present, focused and capable of responding to the directions from the prefrontal neocortex of the brain.

Adaptability is the most crucial aspect for the body's survival. It is critically important in today's world of environmental toxicity, excess stimuli and restlessness. If your matrix cannot adjust and adapt quickly to changing circumstances, this will cause strain on the neuromuscular and organ systems. If your matrix fibers cannot quickly adapt their relationships, when you reach in a new direction or try a new type of food, your system might react with tendon strains and indigestion, respectively.

The three dimensions described above create our resilience, resistance to disease, coping capacities, interconnectedness and balanced relationship to the environments we live in. This foundation of health affects the qualities of the fascial matrix, just as the quality of that matrix impacts our degree of health.

The structure, rhythm, conductivity and boundaries that create the qualities of the living matrix, bridge the cells, tissues and systems of the body into a coherent relationship of continual support, communication and exchange. When these aspects are enlivened, they give us the optimum ability to live and thrive in our ever-changing world.

The qualities of the matrix can either inhibit or enhance the body's internal networks of spatial relations, of which there are three kinds: (1) *enteroception*, in which cells sense where they are in relation to the rest of the internal organs; (2) *proprioception*, in which cells perceive their position, movement and equilibrium in relationship to their surroundings; and (3) *exteroception*, in which cells sense the biosphere, i.e., the entire world surrounding and permeating our planet. The matrix plays an integral part in all three of these relationships. When the matrix is coherent, the body's internal and external relationships are continually informed.

The qualities of the fascial matrix are influenced by the functional needs of the surrounding tissues. The quantity of microfibrils and collagen fibers, cells and molecules, and ground substance varies in relationship to the functional needs in an area as well. The shifting of connections between microfibrils, the arrangement of collagen fibers, the viscosity of ground substance, and the coherence in the field determine the fascial qualities we will be exploring.

The qualities of the fascial matrix determine the shape, space and form of the body, the interrelationship between the layers, and the conductive capacity of the matrix.

The abilities of the fascial matrix to transfer waves and rhythms into cells, slide and glide among organized tissues, and complexify the microfibril connections are determined by the qualities listed below, all of which will be explored in depth in the chapters to follow.

QUALITIES OF FASCIA	
Density/Fluidity:	Gel/Sol, Resistance/Resilience
Slide and Glide:	Mobility/Motility, Stickiness/Slickness
Conductivity:	Dispersion/Coherence
Layering/Compartmentalization:	Interrelationship/Isolation
Suspension:	Buoyancy/Compression
Coherence:	Liquid Crystalline Matrix
Balanced Reciprocal Tension:	Suspension + Coherence
Inertial Patterns:	Isolated, low conductive areas

CHAPTER 3
DENSITY/FLUIDITY

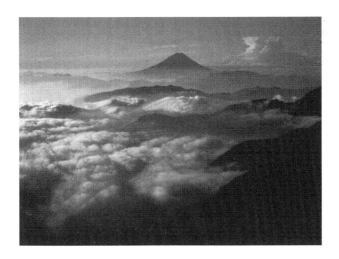

After sunset, a thick mist descends upon the mountain valley. The mist is dense, opaque and full of mystery. At first the shapes of trees, pathways, homesteads and landscaped hillsides gradually begin to recede from view, then suddenly vanish altogether as the mist thickens. Are the footprints of life gone, no longer marching through time? Or are they simply removed from the view of the observer?

Water is a mystery of unfathomable proportions. Each molecule of water in the mist is suspended in the air, careful not to engage with the others, careful not to be drawn into the chains of water that make creek, river, lake and ocean.

Density—like the mist in the mountains—descends into the body as the changes of temperature, the challenges of movement and inactivity, the pressures and tensions and forces of gravity determine the structure of the fascial matrix. The shapes of organs and muscles disappear in the thickening of fascia. Gravity pulls at our shape and movement, just as it pulls at the moisture cooling down at sunset. The changes from day to night, and from movement to stillness, create a rhythm of density and fluidity in the biosphere, as well as in the body's fascial matrix.

During our embryonic development, the pressure and tension of cells reproducing create the variance of density in our fascial collagen fiber makeup. Denser layers of fascia develop around the spine, across the buttocks and down the side of the thigh. When we begin to interact with gravity as an infant, developing movement patterns of sitting, crawling, walking and reaching, we create more longitudinal fibers in legs and arms, while creating hooks around bones and denser matting for stability and support. As we age and grow, layering trauma, injury, overuse and repetitive movement, our fascial matrix increases its density responding to our gravity-held experience.

These changes are also seen on a fractal level within the matrix of the microfibrils. With repetitive movements and habitual lifestyles, the ability to form and inform, as well as to connect and disconnect between the microfibrils, becomes static and limited. The microfibrils pull together to support the repetitive habits creating a thicker, denser matrix.

Like the mist in the valley, the density of the fascial matrix is determined by the temperature, pressures and movement of fluid. And like the mist in the valley, the matrix pulls together and dissipates in response to changes in fluid coherence and suspension.

Let's take a moment now to explore the density and fluidity in your body as it responds to warmth and diverse movement.

---

density – **The distribution of a quantity (as mass, electricity or energy) usually per unit of space (as length, area or volume).**

EXPLORATION 6: FINDING OUR LAYERS OF DENSITY

Find a comfortable position and let your body relax and settle into the space around you. Notice the sensations of heavy and light in your body. Feel the areas of heaviness and notice there size and shape. Notice where you can sense the different layers of the body and where you cannot differentiate. Notice where you feel space or suspension and where you feel compression or thickening. Notice where the contrasting sensations of density and buoyancy meet in your body.

Begin to move your internal matrix slowly by pulling gently away from the torso with the shoulder, noticing where the matrix you are pulling glides and where it resists. Notice how the dense areas move with lots of tissue, resisting the glide between them. Notice the way gliding tissue moves around dense tissue. Move the matrix in different directions to find a denser area.

When you find a dense area, begin to move the internal matrix within it. Start at the superficial layer, gliding and streaming back and forth, allowing the superficial fascia to move freely.

Focus on the deeper density layers and move the internal matrix in slow micro-movements back and forth in all directions from the middle of the density.

Go back to stillness and notice how the dense area has changed, and how it has softened. Move to other dense areas to explore their resistance and movement.

Gently glide your internal matrix, integrating the dense and buoyant areas.

WHAT CREATES DENSITY IN THE FASCIA?

Density is created in the structure of the fascia through the organization and arrangement between the microfibrils and the organized water and the viscosity of the ground substance. When the microfibrils are compressed for long periods of time, they begin to stick together, giving no room for the conductive water channels. Thus, when we are sedentary for long periods of time, the ground substance thickens and increases the density and immobility of the fascia.

Density develops naturally in areas that need more stability and overdevelops in areas of overuse, injury or repetitive movement. When I work with a client who has a frozen shoulder, I glide the matrix in many directions around the shoulder joint, freeing up the compressed microfibrils and drawing in water to organize around them.

Density gives strength and support to an area as a response to the pressure and force of weight or gravity. The collagen fibers may align longitudinally to create support for vertical movement, or they may align multi-directionally for circular movement. The microfibril/water matrix may be more complex in areas of greater movement and less active in areas of limited movement. The normal variations in the quality of density within the body supports movement patterns we use in everyday activities. When we walk, the matrix pulls its arrangement of microfibrils into a long line at the side of the leg around the illiotibial tract. The matrix around the quadriceps muscles on the front of the thigh is more diverse in its complexity to allow for more minute variations of movement.

Density varies daily with temperature changes in the body and within the rhythms of movement and stillness. When we are sedentary and still, the viscosity of our ground substance begins to thicken and the movement between microfibrils is reduced. But as we move, the viscosity lessens to allow for greater glide and microfibril movement. This thickening of ground substance increases with age, which accounts for some of the stiffness we feel with aging.

Density increases in the fascia with trauma, injury, surgery, overuse and repetitive movement. This is due to the rearranging and binding of collagen fibers through crosslinking, which reduces the rearranging of microfibril connections and the amount of organized water between them. Some fascia will thin out due to chronic dehydration. Other fluid system disorders like fibromyalgia can cause irritation in the microfibril/organized water matrix, bringing pain when moving. If you have areas of limited range of motion or an area of numbness or lack of sensation, these may be caused by increased density in your matrix.

When density increases in an area of the matrix, it isolates that area from the information flow of the organism. Sometimes this isolated area creates its own separate flow; we refer to this as an *inertial pattern*. As I work with density in the body, I am always looking for inertial patterns and spending time to reconnect them to the whole matrix. When these inertial patterns persist, they create a space for disease and degeneration to occur.

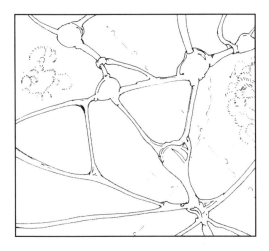

Fig. 11 Healthy Matrix

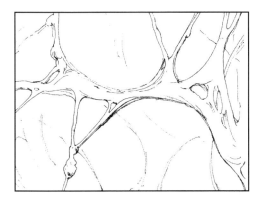

Fig. 12 Dense Matrix

WHAT CREATES DENSITY IN THE FIELD?

Density is created in the field when conductive pathways in the fascial matrix are reduced. When microfibrils shift connections in diverse and complex ways, they maintain an integrated webbing of conductive pathways for the wave patterns to pulsate through, making the conduction strong and consistent. When the microfibrils pull together, reducing the conductive water pathways, the fascial matrix thickens, and this increase of density reduces the flow of information. The field becomes dense with reduced potency and wave motion. In longitudinal density, the conduction becomes stronger in the vertical lines, decreasing the flow of information in all other directions. In multidirectional density, conduction becomes stronger in the area and isolates the area from the wave motions of the integrated body.

When isolated areas develop through injury, overuse and repetitive movement, they create their own field of conductivity—again, an inertial pattern. The integrated conductive field of the body moves around the inertial pattern, cutting off communication and information to the area. This isolated area is the area in your body that aches and throbs when you are still, creating its own expression separate from the functioning of the whole body.

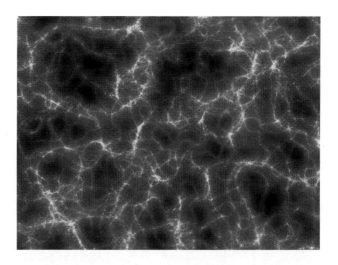

Fig. 13 Protrayal of HealthyFieldMatrix

GEL/SOL

The variation of density in the daily rhythm of the body is partly determined by the gel/sol of the ground substance as we go from inactivity to movement. When we move our bodies the ground substance begins to warm (*sol*), which allows for movement between the microfibrils. It stimulates the organizing of water between the microfibrils and creates buoyancy and suspension in the matrix. When we are sedentary, on the other hand, the ground substance hardens (*gel*) and reduces the ability for the fascial matrix to hold its dynamic relationship between the microfibrils and water. This can lead to over stabilization in the fascial matrix with the microfibrils gluing together and reducing the conductive pathways. Diverse movement can enliven the fascia back to *sol*, keeping it ready to adapt, shift and change with the external and internal inputs. So, start moving in diverse ways and get up from your chair repeatedly: walk backwards, swing your arms behind you, or dance a spiral to warm and open your matrix.

RESISTANCE VS. RESILIENCE

As creatures of habit, we tend to repeat movement patterns and narrow our movement sequences to the tasks we are performing. Injury, trauma, surgery and inertial patterns (isolated areas) limit our range of motion, narrowing the ability of the fascial matrix to adapt, shift and change. The fascial matrix creates holding points to resist the push and pull of gravity, further restricting range of motion. This resistance increases density and thickens the layers of the fascial matrix in the area. The collagen fibers over-stabilize and the microfibrils pull together, reducing the organized water around them.

As the density of the fascial matrix becomes more permanent from the repetition of movement patterns over time, more microfibrils bind together. Through crosslinking and the effects of hyaluronic acid (healthy amounts create slickness, too much creates binding), these areas become dense, isolated and resistant to the fluid movement surrounding it. The fascial matrix can no longer glide and shift its reciprocal balance, creating friction and increase energy use. The body begins to resist moving instead of bounding forward. We feel weak and fatigued, unable to move with ease or without effort. This resistance can have a numbing, pulling or knotted sensation. The tissues feel hard and tough when palpated, not giving way to the pressure of touch or the warming through movement.

When the fascial matrix is healthy and resilient, it feels buoyant, gliding and supporting diverse movement. The fascia is able to engage and disengage the microfibrils, drawing water to organize between them as a response to pressures, tension, shift of weight and conductive inputs. When the collagen fibers shift in response to movement, they return to their original buoyancy and relationship to neutral when the movement is completed.

THICKNESS VS. SPONGINESS

The thickening of areas in the matrix compresses the microfibrils and reduces the spaces filled with organized water. The fibers in the thickened area are glued together with no conductive pathways in between and lose their conductive capacity. The rest of the integrated matrix has to move around the dense area, isolating it. More push and pull is required for muscles to contract, increasing the amount of energy needed for neuromuscular movement. The tough, dense, hardened matrix has no glide or movement, only friction and resistance. When you become fatigued after walking to your car, for example, or find it hard to get up out of a chair, your thickened matrix is part of what is inhibiting you.

When fascia is healthy and enlivened, it feels like a sponge, giving way to pressure and returning to normal when that pressure is released. You can see this when you press your finger to your thigh. It has a buoyant quality, giving way to pressure at first until it reaches its tautness, where it holds, then returning to its normal density when pressure is released. The microfibrils are suspended between organized water, allowing them to shift their connection, conduct through their network and redistribute fluid throughout. Pressure and movement initiate the shifting of matrix connections, giving up fluid to take up the pressure or change in gravity, then replenishing the fluid when the movement is complete. This sponginess and buoyancy can be felt in movement, where the fascia spreads and glides to a point, then holds and supports, maintaining a balanced tension to gravity.

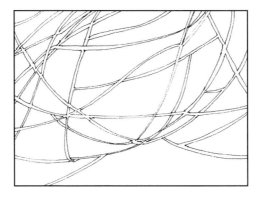

Fig. 14 Spongy Matrix

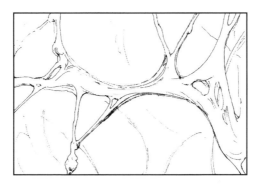

Fig. 15 Thicker Matrix

DENSITY VS. FLUIDITY

The qualities of density and fluidity in healthy fascial layers vary according to the structural variations within the tissue, the functional needs of the areas, pressure and tensions on the tissue, and the effects of movement on the tissue. These qualities shift and change with the viscosity (*gel/sol*) of the ground substance, the diversity of movement in the body and the conductive capacity of the body.

When these qualities become thickened and hardened through the inputs of our lives, they reduce the adaptive, potent, conductive capacity of the fascial matrix. An enlivened fascial matrix shifts and changes its density and fluidity to account for input and movement, while an impaired fascial matrix resists and recoils against input and movement.

DENSITY EFFECTS:

- Conductivity
- Adaptability
- Shape and form
- Level of functioning
- Balanced reciprocal tension
- Vitality and potency
- Energy levels

EXPLORATION 7: PALPATION OF DENSITY

Take a piece of potters clay, modeling clay or clay from your garden. Feel its density and the lack of penetration when you compress it. Continue to press and roll the clay, feeling how it begins to soften as your hands warm it. Clay, like the fascia, can also be affected by the pressure of your hands; the clay particles begin to line up together. As the particles begin to connect, feel how the texture of density begins to change and how you can now feel buoyancy and sponginess in the clay.

Now take a thick sponge and fill it with water. Gently press on the sponge and feel it give way as it releases water. Notice when it resists your pressure. Notice how it comes back to its previous size when you release your pressure.

Feel the sensations of density and sponginess still recorded in your hands.

DENSITY IN INERTIAL PATTERNS

As we age and gather experiences in our fascial matrix, it shapes and forms around those experiences. The collagen fibers align and gather in response to our life's history. When our life is filled with diverse movement and new directions of input, our microfibrils are ready to form and unform with our organized water in diverse, complex arrangements. Thus, our fascial matrix can be said to contain a diverse and complex memory. This memory appears to be held in the crystalline formations of organized water and in the hydrogen surfaces of the microfibrils. This is why we refer to the matrix as a *liquid crystalline matrix* (see Chapter 10 for more details).

Nevertheless, most of our lives are filled with repetitive movement, created by habitual, tedious forms of daily activity and exercise. These habits of the body become ingrained in the memory of the fascial matrix, holding the microfibrils in compression, with limited water between them. The body holds these memories by crosslinking fibers, hardening ground substance and drawing more fibroblasts to the area to build more microfibrils.

This isolated dense tissue creates an inertial pattern in the body. The inertial pattern has its own pulsation separate from the signature wave of the organism. The nourishment in such areas is reduced and the ability to detoxify is diminished. The vitality and potency also becomes low, and such areas can deteriorate over time, leaving an opening for toxins, microorganisms and disease to enter.

By working with diverse movement, gliding the fascial matrix and activating the microfibril/organized water relationship, we can reconnect the inertial pattern into the integrated whole matrix.

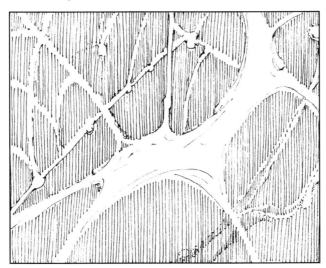

Fig. 16 Inertial Pattern in Matrix

EXPLORATION 8: FINDING OUR INERTIAL PATTERNS OF DENSITY

Find a comfortable position lying down. Relax and settle in. Bring your awareness to your body. Find an area of stiffness, discomfort, pain or density. Notice its size and shape. Notice where its center is located, as well as the edges of the density. Feel the internal matrix that holds this area.

Move the superficial fascia that surrounds the area slowly and notice how it moves around the area of discomfort. Let your movement begin to glide over the area of discomfort. As you move the matrix gently and slowly back and forth, feel how it changes from a sticky, choppy movement to a gliding, fluid movement. Feel when the matrix layer frees itself from the inertial pattern, gliding independently from it.

Focus on the center of the inertial patterned area, and notice how it has its own wave and movement patterns. Initiate a movement in and out from the center of the inertial pattern in multiple directions. Glide through the center of the inertial pattern, out past its boundaries. Then begin to bring it back into the movement pattern of the whole matrix.

Come back to stillness and notice how the area of density has changed.

EXPLORATION 9: FLUID MOVEMENT

(See Gliding the fascia in Self Practice, pg. 214 for more description and illustrations)

Find a comfortable place to lie down on your back, arms above you, and settle into your body. Bring your awareness to your internal matrix.

Initiate a small, slow, gliding, wavelike motion from your right hip down the leg to the feet. Let the foot gently pull that motion to it. Notice how deep it penetrates, how it pulsates through the layers, and when it speeds up or goes around an area. Keep your focus on the fluid internal movement at it goes from each hip and leg into the feet.

Initiate a slow, gliding, internal movement from the torso out one arm. Then do the same with the other arm, and then up through the head. Let the hands and head gently pull the motion to them. Notice how the wavelike movement shifts and changes as you glide the layers of matrix from the center out to the fingers, as well as the top of the head. Stay focused on the fluid movement.

When the movement becomes forced or jerky, relax, change direction and reinitiate the glide in the matrix.

Pause. Notice the way the fluid movement has informed your tissues.

Now let your body glide with fluid movement and pulsate on its own. When it slows or stops at an area, let it choose where to change direction. Let your mind be present in awareness without directing.

If you find the movement beginning to speed up, purposefully slow it down. If it is too slow, give an impulse of wave to move it.

When the body comes to stillness, relax and feel the different sensations in your internal matrix.

As you sit up and go about your day, remind your body of its internal gliding nature and how it supports your movement through space with gliding movement.

MOVING THE FASCIAL MATRIX

Initiating gentle gliding movements that create tautness in the fascial matrix—but not a stretch in the muscle—prepares the fascial matrix to unwind, opening and reconnect inertial patterns and isolated areas. This allows for greater complexity in the microfibril/organized water relationship.

Once the tissue is warmed, open and gliding, we can allow the fascial matrix to move us. By shifting weight, changing our relationship to gravity and creating pressure in different areas, we can stimulate the fascial matrix to slowly shift and change as we follow its gliding movements. As we move effortlessly and with ease, we increase the complexity, vitality and potency of the liquid crystalline matrix and begin to integrate the whole body's conductive system.

With each exploration that moves the internal fascial matrix, (1) we reduce the ability of our habitual patterns to create inertial patterns, (2) we increase our body's ability to respond to external and internal inputs, (3) we increase our range of motion and (4) we bring more ease to the body in motion. If you make a practice of this fluid movement, you will move toward optimizing your health and well-being.

EFFECT OF TOUCH ON DENSITY

When you penetrate the fascial matrix layers with pressure, pull, glide and release, you warm the ground substance and activate the microfibril/organized water to shift and change. Then, as you continue to glide in multiple directions within the denser areas, the microfibrils reconfigure, organizing water into conductive pathways and reconnecting them to the body's integrated crystalline matrix. As the microfibrils shift their dense configuration, they begin to allow for greater penetration, and you can feel the spring-like sponginess return to the area.

When you contact the fascial field where density has created inertial patterns of conductive movement, you can create a conductive flow on either side of the inertial pattern, reconnecting the microfibrils in the dense field. As the inertial pattern reconnects to the integrated matrix, the signature wave pattern of the body conducts and revitalizes the conductive pathways.

Where there is a thinning or stringy quality to the matrix (usually from de-hydration) you can use pressure and release to organize water back in between the microfibrils, restoring the buoyant sponginess of the fascial matrix. When we apply pressure to the fascial matrix, the pressure stimulates the + and − ions in the microfibril structures to align, bringing more charge to the fascial matrix. The microfibrils realign from their charged ends and rebuild the information network. This is known as the *piezoelectric effect*. It can be felt in the tissue as it shifts from being dense and resistant to being buoyant and spongy, and it can be felt in the field as a rich pulsation throughout the body.

---

piezoelectricity – **Electricity or electric polarity due to pressure, especially in a crystalline substance (as quartz).**

EXPLORATION 10: FEELING THE PIEZOELECTRIC EFFECT ON THE MATRIX

Lie on your back with your arms out to the sides. Relax and feel the floor underneath you. Breathe into the floor. Let your arms glide up toward your head very slowly while keeping the back of your arms on the floor. Feel the support and pressure of the floor as you glide your arms around the side of your body. Feel the matrix shifting as you move your arms. Feel the scapula adjusting to your movement.

When your arms are above your head, let the back of your hands and arms press lightly against the floor. Now release the pressure and, clasping your hands together, slowly raise your arms off the floor and up to the front of your body.

Next, bring your hands down over your heart, gently pressing the sternum. Unclasp your hands and let them slowly open up. Feel the piezoelectric effect of buoyancy and lightness in your arms.

Bring your arms back down to your sides and notice the effect of piezoelectricity in your bioelectric matrix.

CASE IN POINT: SHIFTING DENSITY INTO FLUIDITY THROUGH MOVEMENT

The body can create density in any area of the body, whether around a muscle, between muscles, around groups of muscles, or in an area of stress and strain. One of the places I often see this density clearly is between the two bones of the forearm, the *radius* and *ulna*. There is a long space between these two bones where the flexors and extensors of the wrist are found along with nerve and blood pathways. These tissues allow the hand to move in multiple directions. The fascial matrix encircles these layers of tissue between the bones, as well as the bones themselves.

When the body increases density between the bones by binding the layers of fascia together, the definitive lines of muscles and bone disappear and the area becomes thick and hard to penetrate. The sponginess of the buoyant matrix is reduced, and the vitality, strength and glide in the forearm are diminished. Such an inertial pattern isolates and disconnects the forearm.

This scenario is commonly seen in clients who use their hands a lot, where stability and endurance are required. Two different clients recently came to me with acute pain and developing weakness in their left forearm. Both of the clients were massage therapists. The increase of density presented differently in them, and they each had other chronic issues as well.

Jane began seeing me for left neck and shoulder pain after a heavy load at her massage practice. She had previously been a dental hygienist and had developed neck pain from that as well. Her discs deteriorated, and she eventually had a neck fusion at C3/C4. After becoming a massage therapist, and doing regular exercises, she was able to be pain free. Then she developed the pain in the forearm and came back to see me. The forearm had developed significant density between the bones and towards the posterior surface. There was no glide between the extensor muscles or under the retinaculum of the wrist. There was also some density in the front and back of the shoulder. We could see by her movements that she had isolated the forearm in her work to protect her neck, and now an inertial pattern had developed.

I began working with Jane in between her forearm, gliding back and forth from wrist to elbow, gliding the layers of fascia between the extensor muscles and on the inside of the bones. I used micro-movements and figure eights at tighter areas, then glided through the areas to reconnect them with the whole fascial matrix. I also worked on the retinaculum, spreading the bones of the wrist and gliding the fascial matrix between them. I worked on the movement of the head of the humerus in the shoulder joint, gliding the fascial matrix in diverse, spiraling motions, reconnecting the fascial matrix back to the torso and upper arm. After working I noticed the movement in Jane's wrist and arm was more fluid, and she reported that the arm felt stronger.

I showed Jane how to glide the tissue herself by holding at one end and rotating the internal fascial matrix in spiral movements. I also taught her to glide the fascial matrix between the bones, opening the different layers. She felt a significant difference in her arm. The next time she came to see me she wanted to work on her neck and occiput, as her forearm was no longer an issue.

Barbara, another client, had been working with me on helping her body rebalance and stabilize so she could continue doing massage. She had an unstable sacroiliac joint on the right side, and she had broken her left wrist as a child. The wrist had not been set correctly and the hand was rotated slightly. Most of her pain, discomfort and weakness was in her right hip and left shoulder. Then, after we had enlivened the hip and left shoulder, Barbara began to have pain and weakness in her left wrist.

Barbara's density in the forearm was on the anterior side of her forearm. The flexors and the matrix surrounding them were bound together from the wrist to the elbow. I worked on the anterior side of the forearm, gliding the layers of fascia between the flexors and beside the bones. I rotated the arm while putting pressure on the tight areas, creating a piezoelectric effect. I moved the wrist in diverse directions while gliding through the fascial layers. I used micro-movements and figure eights in small, tight areas and at the attachments. I spread the retinaculum while she slowly flexed and extended the wrist, gliding the tendons free. I finished by gliding from forearm to shoulder.

Barbara learned how to glide her forearm's fascial matrix and use internal movements to keep it open. She used diverse fluid movements of rotation and spiral to bring more complexity to the microfibril/organized water matrix and to enhance conductivity.

After the session, Barbara's wrist was greatly improved, and it didn't cause her any more issues for a number of months. As we continued to work on her instabilities and compensational patterns, the wrist pain and weakness would surface at times, needing to be enlivened back into the whole matrix.

CHAPTER 4
SLIDE AND GLIDE

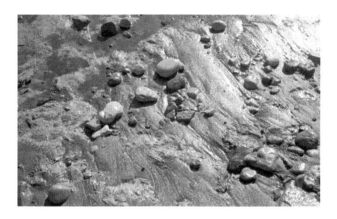

Earth and water are a powerful combination that configures many textures, layers and densities of space, movement and form. When earth is hard clay with particles so close together that water has a hard time penetrating, the water runs off the surface and leaves a slick sheen on the clay. But when the clay is penetrated by water, it begins to expand, its density is reduced, and the clay becomes more pliable. When even more water is added, the clay becomes sticky and the form of the earth changes. When the quantity of water becomes too much for the earth to hold, the clay particles separate and the medium becomes a brown soup spreading out into the space around it.

When earth is sandy, with large crystalline particles, it creates space within it where water can easily travel. As sand becomes saturated with water it pulls together as its crystalline structure allows for conductive flow and is soft and pliable. When there is more water than the holding capacity of the crystalline sand can handle, the water runs through the earth particles, creating depressions in the sandy soil.

When earth is a combination of particles ranging from crystalline sand to tiny particles of clay, and when water penetrates it, you see many different textures and forms arise, including clods of earth, ravines, crevices, mudslides, muddy waters and quicksand.

The texture of the fascia is similar to the combination of earth and water on the planet. When the ground substance and microfibril/organized water matrix in the fascia are hard and compressed, there is little movement or interchange between the fibers and the waters. The fascia is dense and immutable, having a great holding capacity and a small moving capacity.

However, when the ground substance and matrix are more fluid—i.e., the viscosity of the ground substance is lower and organized—then water is organized between the microfibrils, and the fascia becomes more pliable and is able to shape and form around pressure and input. With this greater ability to move and change, the fascia is able to slide and glide within the system while still giving support to form and function. I experience this as an overall fluidity of movement, and the sense that my moving body is buoyant with energy, capable of moving and expressing itself in any way I might want.

When the ground substance remains sticky or the microfibrils are compressed and the crystalline nature reduced, the fascia sticks to the tissues around it and creates friction, reducing its capacity to shape and form around function.

Like earth and water, the quantity and quality of the building blocks of fascia determine the mobility, motility, mutability and slide and glide of the tissue system.

EXPLORATION 11: FINDING OUR SLIDE AND GLIDE

Lying on the ground facing up, let your body rest and settle, letting go into the support of the ground. Focus on your internal matrix and feel it move in waves inside the skin of your body. Let your mind rest and imagine your moving matrix.

With one of your extremities, take up the slack in the internal matrix by slightly pulling away from the torso with a hand or foot, gently gliding from the fingertips or toes to the shoulder or hip. Feel how the superficial fascia glides over the deeper layers. Keep tautness to the fascia and glide back and forth between the shoulder and fingers, hips and toes. Let the glide go deeper into the middle layers of fascia around muscles, bones and organs, by increasing the tautness. Now let the matrix glide on its own, relaxing into the initiation, movement and completion of a glide. Notice the tendency of the glide to spiral and change direction.

Return to stillness and notice the sensation changes in the tissue.

WHAT CREATES SLIDE AND GLIDE IN THE FASCIA?

In order for the body to move continually and with ease, the fascial matrix must be able to shift and move, to glide over the tissue layers, and to respond to the myriad activities of the body. These activities include all of the small internal ripples of the functioning body, as well as our daily movement through space. Our heart beat, breath, cranial rhythm, and deeper, slower tides pulsate through the organized water between the microfibrils, gliding the vibration into our cells. Without this conductive pathway, the movements would create friction as they pulsate. This friction would disperse significant heat and energy, pushing and pulling tissue layers, and increasing the amount of energy needed to move inside and through space.

Moving through space, our muscles contract all or some of their fibers in order to move the bones. The fascia must allow fibers and different muscles to glide over each other in order to move efficiently. This fluidity is gained through the secretion of *hyaluronic acid*, which lubricates the surfaces it lays between. This allows the muscles to work efficiently and glide without friction. Hyaluronic acid helps create the slide and glide between fascia and muscle, along with the viscosity of the ground substance and the complexity of the microfibril/organized water structure.

The slick, wet, fluid nature of the fascia can vary due to different activities, injuries, trauma or restriction. It can vary from a state of stickiness that irritates and creates friction with movement, to a state of slickness that glides smoothly over layers of tissue. With injury, overuse, trauma or immune disorders, the fascia can become fixed and rigid, pulling along all that it touches, creating irritation and overstimulation in the area being moved. The ground substance in such cases may be sticky and grainy, giving a resistance to the movement requiring more energy to move. The microfibril/organized water matrix may be compressed and unresponsive. This friction, irritation and resistance can restrict the flow of blood, lymph and nerve impulses, creating an inertial pattern (in an isolated area).

On the other hand, when the fascia is slick and wet, allowing for smooth movement between layers and tissues, all the systems of the body are enlivened and caressed as the living organism moves. These ripples of movement help to calm the nervous system, stimulating the healthy parasympathetic nervous system to engage in supporting the gliding, free-moving, enlivened body. I find when my matrix is fluid and free, I am calm and relaxed, with my energy stable, constantly restoring itself as I move through the day.

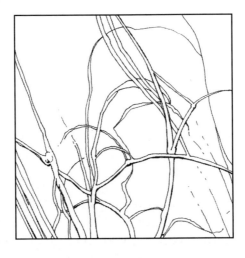

Fig. 17 Fluid matrix

EXPLORATION 12: LUBRICATING THE SURFACE OF FASCIA

Lying in a comfortable position, relax and settle into your body. Focus on the internal matrix. Feel its texture and buoyancy.

Focus your attention on the muscles in your upper arm. Find the part of the matrix that surrounds muscle fibers. Begin to glide the matrix surrounding the muscles, taking up slack by gently moving your hand away from the arm until you feel the tautness in the upper arm. Now glide the matrix by continuing to gently draw the arm down. Let the matrix glide slowly and evenly down the arm muscles. Next, glide back up the arm by gently pulling the matrix with the shoulder. All of these movements happen inside the arm. They are subtle and very small. Feel the glide becoming more fluid. Engage other layers by increasing the depth of the glide.

Glide other parts of the matrix in the leg, hip or torso. Glide until you feel a change in lubrication and a depth of fluid movement. Come back to stillness and feel the new sensations in your body.

HYALURONIC ACID

Hyaluronic acid is a substance that is secreted by the fascia as a lubricant between the fascia and the tissue systems of the body. When hyaluronic acid is secreted at a balanced level, it increases viscosity and glide. But if there is significant strain, injury, compression or overuse, the fascia increases its production of hyaluronic acid beyond its slickness, which can lead to the binding collagen fibers and ground substance and the creation of a thick, sticky surface. Adhesions can then develop, where cohesion between fascia and muscle reduces range of motion, causing pressure and pain to the nerves in the area.

This thickening creates a barrier and increases the acidic nature of the area. Applying heat and raising the pH can decrease the thickening and soften the sticky surface. By moving and gliding the internal matrix in the area, one can draw water back between the microfibrils and bring back the spongy nature to the matrix.

WHAT CREATES SLIDE AND GLIDE IN THE FIELD?

Within the energetic field of fascia, the wave pattern's ability to glide through the fascial matrix of fibers is determined by the strength of the conductive pathway and the complexity and mutability of the microfibril/organized water relationship. This conductive matrix, when changeable and interconnected, creates a consistent container inside which internal pulsations can glide freely. As the microfibrils form and unform the conductive pathways of water, they excite water molecules to align and create a coherent domain. This domain allows the pathways to capture the signature wave of the body and pulsate it through the conductive matrix. The complexity and interconnectedness of this coherent domain determines the strength of the field. This gliding, pulsating capacity allows for greater potency, conductivity and exchange. With sufficient awareness, you can actually feel this as you are dancing or moving and your body fills and empties, ebbs and flows, and glides through space with ease. Give your body the opportunity to move in this way and you will experience the aliveness of your matrix.

When the microfibrils are compressed and anchored to give extra strength to a repetitive motion, it lessens the conductivity and information exchange in the whole system. Conductivity is restricted when there is dehydration, compression or an inertial pattern in an area. You have probably felt this in areas of your body where there is pain when initiating movement or moving past your limitations. By initiating slow, gentle, gliding movements you can decrease these restrictions.

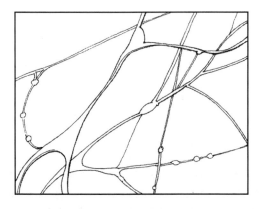

Fig. 18 Shifting Conductive Pathways

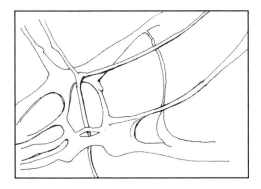

Fig. 19 Restrictive Conductive Pathways

VARIANCE OF SLIDE AND GLIDE

The fascia varies in structure and in its ability to slide and glide, determined by the balance between support, stability and movement. As we move and create rhythms in our lives, we also shift and change the structure of the fascia to meet our needs. The quality of slide and glide—including length and diversity of glide—can support the body in its everyday movements and its relationship to gravity, as well as create a memory pattern of glide and resistance that fits our own habits. When we reach out our arms to draw something to us, our matrix glides in the opposite direction to maintain reciprocal tension, suspending us in gravity. This opposite glide becomes a memory in the matrix so that it can be the stabilizer in this repeated action.

As we develop from a newborn to a fully formed adult, installing the movement patterns of sitting, standing and walking, we build thicker layers fascia to respond to the need for support in the back, buttock and outer sides of the legs. We create cross diaphragms at the shoulders, solar plexus and hips in order to create stability and support. These areas have more collagen fibers connected in a multidirectional webbing of support. These areas have a lowered ability to slide and glide in all directions, allowing for shifts in balance but stabilizing to give support and containment.

Where we have more diverse movement capacity, such as in the shoulders and extremities, the matrix of collagen fibers arrange along the movement patterns needed in those areas. You can palpate those patterned lines in the legs and arms as bands of gathered fibers that support and hold the legs in walking, and the arms in reaching.

Slide and glide varies due to function, ability and need. It also varies due to compression, dehydration, overuse and repetitive movement. When we are sedentary and don't move, our slide and glide is reduced as our ground substance hardens and the microfibrils reduce their need for complexity.

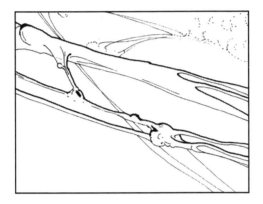

Fig. 20 Repetitive movement and Overuse binds matrix

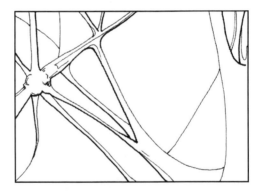

Fig. 21 Complexity of fibers keeps matrix mobile

STICKINESS VS. SLICKNESS

The viscosity of the ground substance and fluidity of the fascial matrix determines mobility and conductive capacity. When the fascia is slick and wet, allowing for smooth movement between layers and tissues, and between microfibrils and organized water, all the systems of the body are enlivened and caressed by the moving living organism. These ripples of movement help to calm the nervous system and activate the parasympathetic nervous system's healthy response to the coherent communication in the whole body.

When the viscosity is sticky and thick, the fascia, unable to slide and glide, begins to bond and harden, reducing its ability to shift with the body's movements and the forces of gravity. This sticky condition reduces the ability of the microfibrils to hold water between them, reducing their conductive pathways and their ability to respond to internal and external inputs.

"It requires more energy for a living system to restrain itself in immobility than to allow movement and shifting…. Tissue that is restrained from change loses its vitality and dissociates from the field of wholeness."

–Bonnie Gintis, DO. *Engaging the Movement of Life: Exploring Health and Embodiment Through Osteopathy and Continuum*, North Atlantic Books, pg. 192.

MOBILITY VS. MOTILITY

Healthy mobility is defined as the body's ability to move in diverse directions. This ability, in turn, is determined by the level of slide and glide in fascial structures. Healthy mobility gives the body that quality of effortless glide and ease of movement between the layers of tissue and through space. When we move from this place, we experience freedom and buoyancy in the body, expressing our inner being in a full and open manner. This mobility determines our range of motion in movement, and the ability for organs to function without interference from surrounding tissues. Mobility allows for smooth, interconnected movement, as well as individual functional movement.

Motility, i.e., the ability to carry vibration through a medium, is determined by the conductive ability of the organized water between the microfibrils.

Motility is the ability of our signature wave to pulsate throughout the matrix constantly. Motility is coherent and interconnected when the waves are free to ripple throughout the coherent domain within the organized crystalline water, replenishing the body's potency. When we come from a space of motility, we are able to take in the impulses of the environment around us and respond to any vibrational demands on us. We can freely express our own vibrational dimensions without inhibition or discord.

When all of our rhythms and vibrations move through this coherent domain, they coalesce into one signature wave, similar to a scalar wave that rises up to vibrate into the field around us. This is what resonates out of our body into the auric field and is our unique signature resonance.

SIGNATURE WAVE AND ELECTROMAGNETIC FIELD

The body is constantly emitting a unified wave pattern that contains all the individual wave patterns, including those from our primitive streak, our emotional, physical and spiritual engagements, and the autonomic activities of our living body. These wave patterns interconnect and become one multidimensional pattern that is our signature resonance. It includes the rhythms of our heartbeat, our breath, our muscles moving, our food digesting, our nerves transmitting. All of these rhythms change their pattern with different internal and external stimuli. This changing wave pattern has constancy in transmission, as it resides in the coherent domain of the organized water pathways between the microfibrils. This excited medium of organized water is like a semiconductor, vibrating its wave patterns continually throughout the matrix.

From the fractal perspective (see Chapter 11), this signature wave can be recognized in each cell, each tissue system, each body, each region, each biosphere, and even our planet. It is a rich, full, resonant wave that constantly connects and informs us. It nourishes us and keeps our body and our planet evolving and changing.

The electromagnetic field that surrounds our planet, our bodies and our cells in the same fractal way as the signature wave is the current that is created by positive and negative ion relationships. In the fascial matrix this ionic lineup is found within the organized water between the microfibrils. The electrons (negative charge) are pulled to the microfibrils by the hydrogen atoms, and the protons (positive charge) are pumped through the enlivened organized water. This is known as the *proton pump* in the matrix. The electromagnetic field is pulsated through this coherent domain of organized water as photons of light that become trapped and weighted in the ionized medium conduct through the matrix). The planet, as well as the cell, has a polar ionic structure that creates an electromagnetic field around them. This is a protective and nourishing field that creates open pathways for wave motion to travel.

EXPLORATION 13: FINDING YOUR SIGNATURE WAVE

Find a comfortable position lying down. Settle into your body and focus on your internal matrix. Let your attention move from the webbing to the collagen fibers, into the microfibrils and the organized water that serves as the conductive pathway. Feel the wave motion and notice how it resonates from any point in multiple directions. Notice how constant the wave motion is in the whole matrix.

Notice your heartbeat and how it is a part of the wave motion in the conductive pathways. Notice the wave pattern of your breath as it pulsates through the conductive pathways. Notice the mid-tide coming from the midline, out in all directions through the microfibrils/organized water matrix. Notice the longer, slower wave patterns as they cycle through the coherent matrix.

Now just relax and feel your deeper signature wave motion. Notice its rhythm as it pulsates in your microfibrils/organized water matrix. Feel the sensation of awareness and consciousness that it provides to your wholeness.

Finally, move from your signature wave to an awareness of your wholeness. Come back to stillness and notice how your sensation of awareness has changed.

EFFECTS OF SLIDE AND GLIDE

- Reduces friction and resistance, freeing up energy
- Allows for individuation of movement
- Allows for a diverse range of motion
- Enlivens and caresses the moving living organism
- Activates the healthy autonomic nervous system
- Mirrors the waves, rhythms and activities of the systems of the body
- Activates changes in the microfibril/organized water matrix

EXPLORATION 14: FEELING THE SLIDE AND GLIDE IN YOUR HANDS

To feel the coherence of slide and glide in your hands, take a can of shaving cream and put a ball of it on one of your palms. Take the other palm and gently press the shaving cream together until your palms are a couple inches apart.

Pull your palms slightly apart to feel the coherence in the cream. From this position begin to slide the palms back and forth, gliding them while holding the full contact of both palms.

Notice that if you pull apart too much, the coherence breaks apart. Notice that if you compress your palms together the cream becomes thinner and the glide is less smooth.

Feel when the glide is evenly sliding the palms back and forth while holding the shaving cream evenly between them. This is what the slide and glide should feel like when you slide and glide healthy fascia.

SLIDE AND GLIDE IN INERTIAL PATTERNS

When the fascial system slides and glides within and around the systems of the body, it balances the nervous system, uses energy efficiently and creates a coherent, interconnected organism. This healthy, fluid internal movement maintains a strong, open mobility and motility.

As creatures of habit, we tend to ask more from certain parts of the body than others. Overuse, injury, dehydration and limited repetitive movement are all factors that shape and form our fascia, ultimately changing what is mean to be an open, interconnected organism. We begin to develop inertial patterns where the slide and glide dynamic has been restricted. When this occurs, the fascia increases its production of hyaluronic acid, creating an acidic, sticky, thick area where the conductive relationship is reduced. Collagen fibers are compressed, and the microfibril complexity diminishes in areas of repetitive use. These areas become separated or insular from the rest of the enlivened body.

With lack of movement, blood and nerve flow, these areas of inertia begin to deteriorate. The nervous system responds with chronic pain signaling, and access is reduced for the immune and endocrine systems. If you have chronic pain in an area of your body that is isolated from the whole matrix, deterioration will continue until you start to glide around and then through the area. Once you initiate a change in the matrix and continue to reconnect it to the whole, your body will be able to heal the tissue that the matrix surrounds and restore nerve, immune and endocrine functions within it.

Inertial patterns maintain their isolation through the thickening of the fascia and the reduction of slide and glide. Motility and mobility are reduced as well. When mobility and motility are weakened and restricted due to compression, dehydration and hardening, the communication and exchange is lessened. All of these factors give rise to areas where the slide and glide and wave patterns go *around* the area instead of through it. This creates some friction and increases the amount of energy needed to move waves and rhythms. The result is a cycle of further deterioration and an enlargement of the area.

When we use touch or movement to increase the slide and glide in our fascia layers, we begin to reduce the areas of inertial patterns. This reorganizes the microfibril/organized water matrix and restores the coherent domain where the wave patterns can flow.

EXPLORATION 15: GLIDING YOUR INERTIAL PATTERNS

Find a comfortable place to lie down and settle into your body. Scan your body for areas of discomfort, stiffness, soreness or lack of sensation. If you already know of an area that is isolated from the whole body, work in that area.

Focus on the internal matrix that surrounds the area. Begin by letting it glide gently from your midline out to the area of inertial pattern you are working with. Notice where it slides and glides evenly and where it sticks and jumps forward, or doesn't move at all.

Now focus on the inertial pattern. Notice the size, shape and depth of the pattern. Glide back and forth around it to feel how it is isolated and does not participate in the slide and glide movements of the matrix. Glide in different directions until you can feel the isolated area responding to the coherent matrix outside of it.

Focus at the center of the isolated area and do tiny micro-glides in multiple directions to open the area from the center out.

Now glide back and forth across the insolated area until it dissolves and reintegrates back into the whole matrix.

Repeat with other areas of concern.

Finish by gently letting the matrix move itself reintegrating the inertial pattern.

EXPLORATION 16: VARIANCE OF GLIDE, MOTILITY AND MO-BILITY

Find a comfortable place to lie on your back. Settle into your body. Focus on your internal matrix. Feel its wave pattern and let your body glide and move to its rhythm.

Initiate a glide from the hip down the leg to the toes and back, by pressing your toes to the floor and up toward your head.

Next, initiate a glide using your heel to bring it down the back of the leg, and using your hip to pull the glide up the front of the leg. Vary the speed of the glide, slowing it down. Notice how much more of the matrix you engage when you slow down. Vary the depth of the glide, noticing the different layers you can engage. Vary the strength of the glide, noticing how you are engaging more of the matrix. Repeat on other leg and each arm.

Come back to stillness and notice the changes in sensation and pulsation in the legs.

Focus on the midline of the body and initiate a glide moving out to the extremities and back. Notice the mobility of the tissues as you glide in and out. Notice how the matrix moves between the other tissue and around organs.

Focus on the midline of the body and find the wave pattern that emerges from the midline and vibrates out to the extremities and back. Notice the strength, rhythm and speed of the wave pattern, feeling the motility of the internal matrix.

Return to the midline and notice the different sensations in the body.

EFFECTS OF TOUCH ON SLIDE AND GLIDE

The ability of the fascia to slide and glide is determined by the body's diverse movement patterns, viscosity of the ground substance, and the complexity of the microfibril/organized water matrix. With the repetitive, habitual nature of our lives, we reduce our slide and glide to the lines of movement we make. So, we can work with the Explorations described above to open the inertial patterns and enliven the fascial matrix and/or use hands-on touch to open more capacity for fluid movement.

When we use our hands to manually glide the fascial layers, the heat from our hands softens the ground substance and gives it more ability to glide. The movement of glide begins to reorganize the microfibril/organized water matrix and increases our mobility and range of motion. As we glide in multiple directions, following the unwinding patterns, we increase the ability of the microfibrils to shift and change as we move and relate to gravity.

When we glide each fascial layer, we give it more complexity and a greater capacity to adapt to input and range of movement. We open up spaces for muscles, bones and organ systems to function, letting our signature wave inform them of the activities of the integrated organism.

To glide the fascial layers, we start by pulling up the slack in the tissue. The superficial fascia has the most slack, so it can shift and change with broad movements through space. As we go to the deeper layers, however, the fascial glide varies. We can use our hands to anchor a layer and then glide it between the tissue systems it is surrounding.

When we glide a fascial layer we create tautness with a two-hand contact, so we can pull and glide the tissue between the two contact points. We slide and glide the tissue back and forth between our hands, increasing the glide within the area between the two points. We shift our hands to change the direction of glide, guided by the unwinding movement of the fascial matrix. We finish by gliding a broader area to reconnect the inertial area to the whole system.

By gliding the fascial layers and reconnecting them to the whole organism, we return the body to an enlivened, connected whole.

EXPLORATION 17: USING HANDS TO SLIDE AND GLIDE PARTNER'S MATRIX

Place hands on either side of the anterior thigh, above the knee and below the hip. Give gentle pressure so you penetrate past the skin.

Create a tautness with the upper hand by pulling away from the lower hand. Gently glide the tissue with both hands towards the hip until you feel it resisting your pull. Pause.

Create a tautness with your lower hand by pulling away from your upper hand. Slowly glide the tissue between your hands downward until you feel the resistance from the upper hand. Pause.

Continue back and forth, gradually gliding more tissue, both longitudinally and deeply.

Glide back and forth between the foot and hip to integrate to the larger matrix.

Repeat this process anywhere on the body to increase the slide and glide in the internal matrix.

CASE IN POINT: DRY EYE, GLIDING THE CONJUNCTIVA

Enhancing the slide and glide of the fascial matrix allows for lubrication, movement and protection for the tissues that are functioning next to the fascial layer. This is true anywhere in the body and can be used to address dryness, friction and irritation in any of our tissue layers. So when I was asked by a client if I could improve a severe case of dry eye when nothing else had worked, I said I would give it a try.

Susan came to see me after she had tried everything for the severe redness and dryness in her eyes. She was constantly blinking and sometimes unable to keep her eyelids open. She had a regiment of putting drops in her eyes and sleeping with goggles to protect them from drying air and other irritation. However, her eyes continued to cause her discomfort, blinking and redness, so she was now wearing the goggles during the day as well. She was not on any prescription drugs that would further cause dryness, and she drank plenty of water.

I first worked on Susan's shoulders and neck to see if there was some pull in the matrix from the areas below her face. Finding some inertial patterns in her neck, I glided the different soft tissue layers in the neck, then did small figure eights around the vertebrae, discs and inter-spinal muscles. After opening and complexifying the matrix of her neck and shoulders, I moved to the head and face.

Working with the matrix on the surface of the head and face, I found some areas over-suspended and some areas over-cohered. I used glide and compression to rebalance the reciprocal tension in the back of the head, around the ears and into the face. I brought the areas back into reciprocal balance, and I could feel the pull of the matrix from the conjunctiva on the surface of her eyes.

Next, I began to work around the orbital bones and top of the nose, using my fingers to glide back and forth from her nose to the outside of her eye socket. When that horizontal part of the matrix opened, I began glided at angles around the eye socket. As these angles opened, I glided deeper into the membranes of the sinuses in the nose and below the eyes. Once the area was open, I used the glide to reconnect it to the matrix in the head and neck.

Susan returned for five more sessions. She reported each time that her eyes felt less irritated, that she could go longer without using the drops, and that her blinking had reduced. By our final session, Susan was no longer using her goggles at all, and she was able to be comfortable all day. When her eyes felt like they were getting dry, she would perform the eye exercises I had given her, moving the matrix in multiple directions, and the dryness would quickly subside. She had additional issues with her neck and upper back that we continued to address, so that the matrix around the conjunctiva would not pull downward or shift the balanced reciprocal tension in her face and head.

She was greatly relieved to be able to see the world again through clear, unblinking eyes.

CHAPTER 5
CONDUCTIVITY

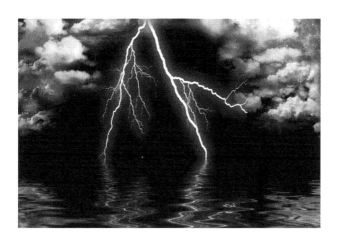

The Earth is surrounded by an electromagnetic field that creates a shield of protection from outer space and keeps other charged fields from entering our atmosphere. Within our atmosphere there are many forces that activate charged particles and create currents of their own. When these static, chaotic forces move into alignment, they sometimes create currents of electricity seen in the sky as lightning. Sometimes lightning is a strong bolt propelled to the ground, and sometimes it meanders horizontally across the sky. Wherever the organized matrix of meteorological patterns allows charged particles to become electricity is where lightning illuminates the sky. It is an amazing sight to watch a matrix build and become a conduit for electrical forces. It is a powerful current that can create fires, split trees in half or take down an entire electrical grid.

As we have seen, the body's fascial matrix that allows our bioelectric field to move and flow, exchanging vibration and information, comes from the microfibril/organized water matrix. The organized water between the microfibrils creates a coherent domain that pulsates our wave patterns through the body and vibrating into our cells.

Sometimes the microfibril/organized water matrix flows in a vertical direction that creates a strong flow up and down the body, as illustrated by the acupuncture meridians. In the cross-diaphragms at the hips, solar plexus and shoulders, the flow is multidirectional, creating more stability. The microfibrils are continually engaging and disengaging with the water that organizes between them, from the time of their arising out of the mesenchyme throughout the life of the organism. When the microfibril/organized water matrix complexifies, engaging and disengaging in diverse and multidirectional ways, it increases the number of pathways that conducts our waves and rhythms. This also increases its contact points to our cells, so that it touches every cell in the body, transferring the wave pattern information to the cytoskeleton of microtubules in the cells.

EXPLORATION 18: FEELING CONDUCTIVITY IN THE BODY

Find a comfortable place to lie down and settle into your body. Turn your focus to the internal matrix and feel its fluid motion. Focus more specifically on the microfibrils and the organized waters between them. Imagine the electrical pulsations that move through this matrix. Now focus on your heartbeat and imagine it pulsating through this matrix. Let that pulsation go and again find the wave motion within the organized water of the matrix.

Let the wave motion pulsate through the microfibril/organized water matrix and then into the cell's cytoskeleton.

Notice the vibration conducting in the microfibril/organized water matrix going in multiple directions, up the body, down the body, from the midline out and in, and spiraling out the extremities. Now come to stillness and notice your new sensations of conductivity in the body.

WHAT CREATES CONDUCTIVITY IN THE FASCIA?

Our matrix of collagen fibers and microfibrils creates the container in which the pulsation of our wave patterns resonate. The organized water that is held within and between these tubular (microfibril) structures is the conductive medium. These tubular structures are created by the fibroblasts, plentiful within the fascial matrix. Fibroblasts use different proteins to connect triads of collagen molecules that bind together to make protein polymer strands of microfibrils. These microfibrils are hollow on the inside, with hydrogen atoms lined up on the inside and outside of the tube. These hydrogen atoms bond with other hydrogen and oxygen molecules to create a H_2O fluid medium within and without the microfibrils. This water organizes its electrons on the surface of the microfibrils, and its protons organize in the middle, creating an electrified coherent domain. The protons dislocate and move up the microfibrils, creating a conductive pulse. This electrified coherent domain traps the electromagnetic resonance of the organism and pulsates it through the matrix.

The microfibrils spiral around each other to form triple helixes of collagen fibers with the organized water between them. In their formation, the ends of the collagen fibers have + and – charges, allowing them to connect end-to-end or twist and turn away from each other. This gives the fibers the capacity to spiral and become like springs, pulling and stretching with movement.

The multiple connections in the microfibril/organized water matrix create a dynamic webbing between and around the tissue layers and organ systems in the body. As our different systems function they vibrate their activity through the fascial matrix. The matrix pulsates this vibration into the microtubules in the cells, maintaining constant contact with every cell in the body. This gives the fascial matrix the ability to record and communicate all the rhythms, movements and exchanges that go on from cell to tissue to external stimuli. This contact and interconnectedness allows the tissues to relate as one alive system.

As the body moves, this movement is transferred through the collagen fibers and microfibril/organized water matrix, informing all the cells in the body. This gives direct immediate information to the systems that move the body, readying them for action. This transfer of information gives the body the ability to move smoothly, efficiently, and with ease. Movement is a dance of relationship, connecting all parts of the system. It is an amazing, diverse, dynamic system that allows us to flow through life physically and energetically.

The protein-based microfibrils shift and change by building or letting go of the organized water between them. They are continually adapting to the inputs into the system through this dance of releasing and binding water into a coherent domain. This can be seen as microfibrils separating, or as droplets of organized water moving down the microfibrils, changing their contact points. These shifts and changes in microfibril relationships come from changes in movement, our relationship to gravity, and functional activities within the organism. As microfibrils shift and change their contact points during activity, they inform the cells of the changes. When the cells shift and change their wave pattern, the matrix informs the others cells of the changes.

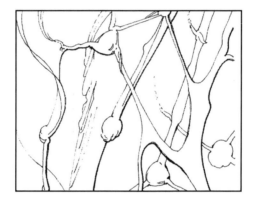

Fig. 22 Matrix of conduction

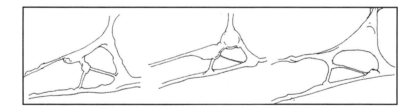

Fig. 23 Organized water moving between microfibrils

WHAT CREATES CONDUCTIVITY IN THE FIELD?

A conductive field is created when organized energy has a medium in which to flow. The conductive field of fascia pulsates our signature wave (organized energy) through the coherent domain of water between the microfibrils. It informs the cells of all the inputs, outputs and exchanges in the body. In order for this field to maintain its coherence, fascia must have a fluid, flexible and stable pathway in which to move the organized energy.

The conductive field of fascia, organized around its embryological, functional and relational energy, supports the structural conductive function of the microfibril/organized water matrix. It brings potent energy, support and relationship to the whole body. This conductive field forms at the first pulsation of the primitive streak and continues to pulsate through the bioelectric matrix throughout the life of the organism. When the field is strong and organized, the body is enlivened, vital and full of potency. This can be felt as a zest for life, springing out of our shoes, or fully experiencing the moment. However, when the field is impeded by disconnection, containment and inertial patterns, the body is weak and open to disease and degeneration. This can be felt as fatigue, loss of appetite for life, or chronic pain and strain in the muscles and tendons.

CONDUCTION VS. DISCONNECT

When the body's microfibril/organized water matrix is complex and diverse, it is able to conduct all of the impulses of the body to the cells immediately through its complex webbing. When the microfibrils are engaging and disengaging with the organized water in complex and diverse ways, the matrix is able to pulsate each new wave into the system. Each layer of pulsation in the body becomes a continuous wave in the microfibril/organized water matrix.

As we shift and change with the inputs from the internal and external environment, the matrix also shifts and changes its conductive pathways to keep the cells informed of these inputs. This ability to shape and form to our internal and external environment creates the coherence and integration that we need to perform complex activities in the world. In our day to day lives, we have to respond to everything from temperature to danger. The nervous system responds to these inputs, while the matrix system informs the cells immediately and automatically without comment. Because the matrix is a coherent field, the cells are informed immediately without the delay of synapses running from afferent to efferent nerve pathways.

When the matrix condenses, solidifies or disconnects, the cells are less informed and unable to adapt and shift to the environmental inputs. The cells become disconnected from the whole body and no longer receive information about the rest of the body. This disconnect, whether in small or large areas, creates an inertial pattern in the area and diminishes the area's vitality and ability to function. The area is no longer a part of the coherent whole, deteriorating and opening up the way for disease. Inertial patterns are the forerunners of diseases in organs, strains and spasm in muscles, and digestive disorders, just to name a few.

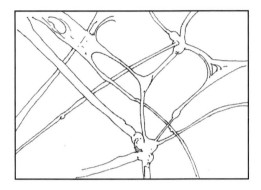

Fig. 24 Matrix beginning to bind together

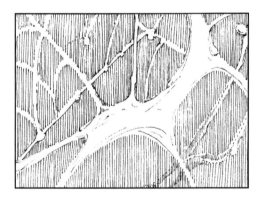

Fig. 25 Solidified part of matrix

COHERENCE VS. DISPERSION

Coherence is the ability to create order and consistency in an ever-changing environment, allowing for continuity and continuous exchange. The fascial bioelectric matrix supports the body's coherent ability to inform individual cells. It also creates an immediate energy loop to allow for efficient, smooth response to the inputs and relationships in the internal and external environments. This fascial coherence is what gives us the ability to feel the interconnected wholeness of the enlivened body, manifesting as a sense of vitality and the feeling that your body is ready for any challenge. In short, our health and well-being are determined by the immediate, coherent exchange of information between matrix and cells.

When our body's bioelectric matrix is impaired, and the inertial patterns of the body don't allow all cells to receive the information needed, this creates pools or eddies of wave pulsations within the microfibril/organized water matrix. This not only reduces the total information exchanged within the body, it also creates an aberrant pulsation that disperses to the surface of the body. We sometimes feel this as a dull achy sensation, where the inertial pattern is pulsating out toward the nerves. This wave interferes with the coherent wave in the integrated part of the matrix, shifting the strong, coherent resonance in this part of the body into a dispersed, disconnected, chaotic field that affects all other body systems.

Have you ever felt as if a part of your body—your forearms for example—were disconnected from the rest of your body? Well, there is a good chance that, on the fascial level, they were disconnected from the coherent wave of your body.

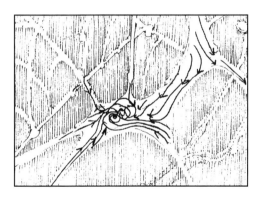

Fig. 26 Inertial flow of energy between microfibrils

MESODERMIC RELATIONSHIPS IN CONDUCTIVITY

From the beginning of life, when the primitive streak moves through the bilaminar disc (formed by ectoderm and endoderm stem cells) and begins the pulsation of life, the mesodermic tissue becomes tuned to our individual resonance and vibration. The tissue continues to pulsate as it shapes and forms the space for our different functioning systems, giving our bodies their ability to perceive, move and respond in life. The fascial matrix is the conductive medium where the continual pulsations of life are linked to the mesodermic essence of curiosity, movement and adaptation.

Fascia connects to all the mesodermic tissues (muscle, tendon, ligament, blood, lymph, etc.) through its embryological memory. Its microfibril/organized water matrix of collagen fibers also connects to the collagen fibers in muscle, tendon and ligament, creating a continual network of exchange within the fascial/musculoskeletal system.

Because the fascial fibers interface with other connective tissues, conduction can spread into other tissues such as ligaments and tendon. When the fascia fibers are spread in many directions, the conduction may spread out in all directions. Where fascia is longitudinal, the conduction will move up the body, aligning with the spine and the midline.

EXPLORATION 19: FINDING YOUR MESODERMIC CONNECTIONS

Find a comfortable position lying down and settle into your body. Focus on your internal matrix. Imagine its structure of round, hollow microfibrils. Feel the pulsation of information as it moves through the organized water in the matrix. Deepen into the stillness until it opens into a very subtle back and forth rocking movement and follow that movement through the matrix.

Shift your awareness to the superficial layers fascia under the skin, and feel its pulsations connecting to the skin and deeper tissues. Shift your awareness to the matrix surrounding the muscles of your thigh. Feel the layers and follow them as they connect to the tendon and bone. Find the deepest layer of fascia surrounding the spinal cord. Feel its layers and follow its connection out into the middle fascia from connection points in the neck, upper spine and lower spine. Now shift your awareness to the microscopic level and find the mesodermic stem cells in your body.

Imagine your are going back in time until you find the stem cells that make up the mesoderm; feel the primitive streak that creates it. Then move forward in time and feel the spreading of connective tissue fibers through the body that create its shape, form and function.

Bring your awareness back to your whole matrix. Notice the different sensations you feel in your body now.

PATTERNS OF CONDUCTIVITY

The fascia conducts all the waves and rhythms within the functioning of the body, all the movements of the body, and all external inputs of pulsation. These waves vary in terms of speed, rhythm and intensity.

The waves and rhythms within the body systems include the heartbeat, breath, cranial rhythm, mid tide and long tide. The fascia also conducts all of the movements and shifts in the centrioles of the cells and the muscular-skeletal movements of the body through space. As we allow the external rhythms of the Earth and other living things into our body, they can pulsate through our bioelectric matrix as well. Whenever there is skin stimulation through touch, temperature or moisture, this resonates through the microfibril/organized water matrix.

Our touch in hands-on work impulses information into the system. We put an impulse into the body from the surface by gently pushing or pulling on the fascia and follow it as it ripples through the body.

These resonant wave patterns differ in pulse, duration and meter. The pulse, a periodic beat equally spaced in time, can differ in its beat, being slow and long as the long tide, or quick and fast as the heartbeat. When the heart beats faster, that changes its wave pattern and all of the cells are aware of this change.

Each beat can also change its duration, i.e., the space between the pulse. The patterns can also vary in meter, i.e., how each beat is accented. These patterns of pulse, duration and meter vary between the different wave patterns, as well as within a specific wave pattern. These differences are pulsated through the tissues of the body and into the cells. When the duration or meter of the heartbeat changes, every cell in the body is aware of the shift and can respond to it. When the duration or meter of the breath changes, the change is felt in every cell so they can respond. These changes are crucial for the cells to maintain nourishment and homeostasis.

Rhythm is the expression of the different pulses of wave movement in the organized waters. The rhythm that is pulsating through this bioelectric field is the signature resonance of the body: a coherent, unified pulsation. The rhythm varies as the patterns change and the cells respond to the new pattern.

The pathway of movement through the bioelectric matrix is determined by the arrangement of the microfibrils. The wave pattern moves out and in at horizontal diaphragms, and up and down at the longitudinal layers around muscles and bones. As the pattern changes, the whole system vibrates differently.

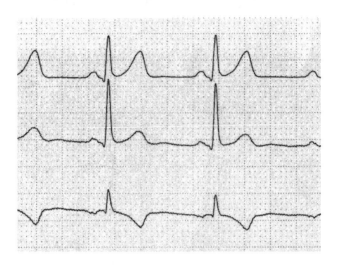

Fig. 27 Heart Rate wave pattern

Normal Adult Brain Waves

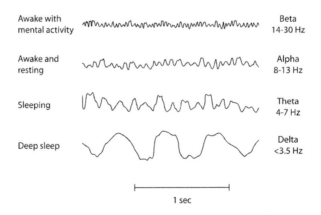

Fig. 28 Brain Wave pattern variance

EXPLORATION 20: FINDING YOUR PATTERNS OF CONDUCTIVITY

Find a comfortable position lying down and settle into your body. Bring your awareness to your internal matrix. Imagine its structure.

Shift your awareness from structure to the waves of energy inside the waters of your matrix. Notice its pulse, duration and meter.

Now begin to differentiate waves patterns. Begin by noticing the heartbeat. Feel how its wave pattern moves throughout the body.

Next, bring your awareness to your breath. Feel how this slower rhythm pulsates throughout the body, moving through the microfibril/organized water matrix.

Bring your awareness to the cranial rhythm, feeling its pulsations rotating around the midlines of your body. Notice how the pulsations spiral out through the body.

Now bring your awareness to the deeper, slower rhythm of the mid tide. Feel how it flows in and out from the midline. Notice the way the pulsations move through the body.

Next, bring your awareness to the very slow pulsation of the long tide. Feel how it moves slowly up the body, pulsating through the organized water.

Finally, bring your awareness back to your integrated signature wave, feeling the waves of heartbeat, breath, cranial, mid and long tide fold into your signature wave.

EFFECTS OF CONDUCTIVITY

- Creates a coherent resonance that protects the body from the external electromagnetic fields
- Connects all the tissues in the body
- Informs all the cells of the shifts and changes in the body immediately and continually
- Creates a medium for connecting and relating to the external resonant environment
- Creates an information matrix to keep all the tissues in the body informed
- Creates a signature wave that reflects our unique individual resonance

EXPLORATION 21: FEELING CONDUCTIVITY IN YOUR HANDS

Begin by rubbing the palms of your hands together to create static electricity between them. Now put palms facing each other a foot away. Slowly bring them together until you can feel the pull, warmth and charge between them. Go back and forth at this point to feel the conductivity as it becomes stronger and weaker.

Next, take a pair of strong magnets, one in each hand. Slowly bring them together feeling the pull as they snap together. Go back to the place where you begin to feel the pull and slowly move them back and forth. Notice the slight push away before they begin to pull strongly together. Hold them at the place where the pull between them can be felt, and notice how that feels in your hands and up your forearm. This is the electromagnetic pull that you can feel in the microfibril/organized water matrix.

INERTIAL PATTERNS IN CONDUCTIVITY

Where there are inertial patterns of compression, disconnection or isolation, the conductive capacity in the area is greatly reduced. Inertial patterns disconnect an area of trauma from the body, dispersing the coherence and reducing or eliminating the information exchange between tissues in that area. These areas continue to become isolated over time, and they are essentially unprotected from internal and external input, reducing nourishment and detoxification, as well as its relationship with the other functioning systems. The microfibrils compress and the organized water within them is diminished, lowering the ionic capacity of conduction. This further deteriorates the area unless the conductive pathways are reconnected to the whole system. When you feel such a disconnect in your body, where the back is solid and disconnected from the legs, it is important to re-enliven the microfibril/organized water matrix to return health and mobility.

Sometimes the wave patterns moving through the bioelectric matrix circle around the inertial patterns. This creates eddies and pools that are separate from the body's signature wave. Sometimes these eddies create their own conductive patterns and flow. These separate, isolated patterns can be seen as a threat to the whole body and further reinforce the isolating, degenerating cycle.

You can sometimes feel these isolated conductive patterns within an area of your body as heat, tremors or circular movement. When they are touched, you can feel the patterns moving within the isolated area, as well as feel the coherent body outside the area moving around them.

EFFECTS OF TOUCH ON CONDUCTIVITY

Because we are all conductive, resonant beings, when we touch another person we connect our bioelectric matrix to theirs. When we make that connection, our individual matrix decides if and how much it wants to connect with the other one. When there is trust and safety, we connect our matrices and become able to listen and respond to each other's conductive pattern.

When we find inertial patterns in the body, where conduction is reduced or a separate wave pattern is created, we can use an impulse to break up the isolated pattern, listen to the pattern, or be a witness to the relationship of the inertial pattern to the coherent pattern.

By bringing new input to the area through our own resonant touch, we can begin the process of opening an isolated area and reestablishing the coherent domain of organized water. A body that is being touched will witness the difference between the two, and all of its systems will begin to listen to the inertial pattern. This brings a conductive dialogue into the tissues and gives them the opportunity to focus on reconnecting their conductive pathways.

With touch, we can open up inertial patterns, shifting the circling conductive pattern, opening the isolated eddies of energy and reconnecting this part of the microfibril/organized water matrix to the whole. This brings coherence, vitality and potency back to the area, allowing the tissue to heal and renew.

Our bodily systems strive to be integrated and interconnected, always trying to reconnect with isolated areas. When awareness is brought to an inertial pattern, this attention can stimulate it to unwind and reconnect. Whether through internal movement or hands-on work, when the body takes the time to unwind an inertial pattern, it is capable of renewing deep levels of degeneration. When this is done regularly, the body learns to notice and reconnect as an inertial pattern begins to develop, helping to avoid their recurrence.

EXPLORATION 22: FINDING CONDUCTIVE INERTIAL PATTERNS ON A PARTNER

Place your hands above an area of discomfort in you or a partner. Slowly move your hands around until they are touching either side of the area. Notice the connection that happens as you engage.

Settle your hands around the area. Feel the coherence (pulling together of any area and its ebb and flow) that is connecting the area outside of the inertial pattern. Let your hands follow that movement.

Now bring your hands over the area of discomfort and settle into its conductive pattern. Notice the difference between the area of discomfort and the surrounding areas of coherence. Feel the heat, pressure or lack of pulsation in the inertial area.

Go back and forth from the coherent pattern and inertial pattern, noticing the difference in the quality and pull.

Find another area of discomfort and repeat the process, bringing awareness to the different qualities of conductivity in the body.

Come back to the first area you found. Repeat the sequence of engagement, feeling sensation and following movement in the surrounding area. Then move hands over the original area of discomfort. Notice how it has changed.

Take your hands off the body and let your partner integrate the new sensations of touch and pulsation.

CASE IN POINT: DISCONNECTED CONDUCTIVITY, EFFECTS OF A HIP REPLACEMENT

Carla came to see me one year after a hip replacement with pain in her replaced hip socket. She had a noticeable limp and was unable to walk very far. She was in pain most of the day and had a hard time finding a position to sleep comfortably. Some days, though, the pain and discomfort would be completely gone, then gradually come back after a few days. She had been to her surgeon and, after evaluating the hip replacement, he had said that her pain was *not* from the surgery. She came to me hoping to find some relief.

Carla lay down on my table, and I began my work. First, when I put an impulse up her leg to the replaced hip, I found that there was no conduction in that whole side. Her left leg and hip were disconnected from the rest of her body and had their own inertial conductive pattern. The opposite side had a lateral conduction with no connection at the horizontal diaphragms. The matrix was completely disconnected in multiple directions, giving no support and exchange of information to the system.

I began my treatment by gliding her right side, where there was some conduction, and enhancing the normal conductive pattern of her body. I slowly worked up the leg, through the hip and up the back. Once the conductivity in her right side was strong, I began to do figure eights at the hips to bring the conductivity into the left side. I continued the figure eights at the ribs and neck. Then I began gliding and reconnecting the left ankle, knee and hip, opening up the conductive pathways of the left leg. I used the glide throughout the leg, gliding from heel to hip, then up the back. I finished by gliding up the spine, anchoring the conductive patterns in the midline.

I saw Carla every week for a month, then every other week for a few more months. Gradually, her conductive capacity in the left side reconnected to the whole matrix, and each week she had less pain, more mobility and was able to walk a longer distance. The matrix around the hip replacement still had some areas where the conduction was not strong, but her body seemed to find a way to compensate. Carla began to exercise and walk more, feeling more stability and coherence when moving.

I continued working with Carla, engaging other issues in her upper body, but always coming back to the left hip to reengage it into the whole matrix. Even though the complexity of the microfibril/organized water matrix is still diminished by the surgery, Carla's body has compensated, finding a way to bring the area back into the integrated whole.

CHAPTER 6
LAYERING/COMPARTMENTALIZATION

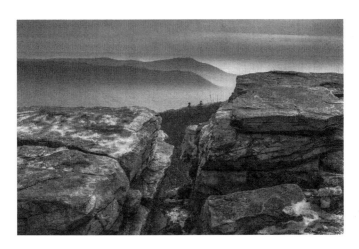

Our planet's history is recorded in its layering of rock and earth. Geologists construct timelines of geological history from these layers. The earliest layers formed to create the Earth's crust around its core of magma. Some layers were formed through the generative forces of earthquakes, uplifts and shifts in the Earth's crust. These forces gave shape and relationship to mineral, water, fire and space. Once the planet's surface was stabilized and the elements began to intermingle, the container for life—i.e., the planet as we know it—was established.

The Earth continues form and reshape in response to both internal and external forces. On the internal level, the plates within the Earth move and shift, creating earthquakes and fissures on the surface. As these forces move, the surface shifts to accommodate them. Surface changes across the land and undersea shape and form from the external forces of wind and water, as well as human interaction. These forces reshape the surface through the wearing away of existing layers, the moving and shifting of layers, and the building of new layers. These changes can happen quickly or over a very long timeline.

The fascia in the body is similarly layered, formed by the mesodermic stem cells. These cells shaped and formed the containers for our organs, tissues and vessels. Once these layers were established in the fetus and a human body was fully formed, a human life entered the world.

Our bodies continue to shape and form throughout life, determined by both the internal and external environment. The fascia slides and glides, shifting its bioelectric matrix to accommodate for movement, growth, reproduction and activity.

The matrix shifts continually to respond to the external and internal influences of nutrients, toxins, movement and contact. The layering of fascia in the body allows the body to maintain its integrity, give organs space to function independently and protect tissues from the external contact with the world. Our layers of fascia vibrate and modulate our bioelectric field throughout the body's internal environment. This vibration extends into the external environment, meeting the bioelectric field of the Earth.

WHAT CREATES LAYERING IN THE FASCIAL STRUCTURE?

The initial layering of fascia within in the body takes place as the embryo develops. Beginning with the primitive streak, when the midline is formed, the push and pull resulting from cell division causes mesodermic stem cells to form pockets and layers that give space for the endoderm and ectoderm to create the digestive system, nervous system and skin. The connective tissue also forms the musculoskeletal connections for support and movement, as well as the blood system for the transporting of nutrients and toxins.

This layering in the fascial structure has a surface layer that is called the "sleeve," which is two layers (superficial and deep) beneath the skin. This sleeve essentially provides shape to our external form. These two layers connect through fibers called *retinacular cutis*. The myofascial layers of fascia surround the muscles, tendons and ligaments, creating functional space. This matrix layer connects to the fascial layers of the periosteum around the bones. The visceral fascia encases the internal cavities of the torso and surround the organs, protecting and giving space for independent functioning. The deepest layer of fascia surrounds the spinal cord and brain, giving space for the cerebral spinal fluid to nourish the nervous system.

The layered structure described above is entirely interconnected, creating a web-like matrix of conductivity within the body. The microfibril collagen fibers are intertwined between the layers, between the fascia and the cells, and between the fascia and muscular/skeletal tissues. These structures create a continuous conductive pathway of organized water that transmits and vibrates information through the body.

Because the webbing of the fascia surrounds each of these tissue systems, it unifies them through the exchange of information it provides. Because of the semiconductor-like ability of the microfibril/organized water matrix, the exchange of information happens much faster than in the nervous system.

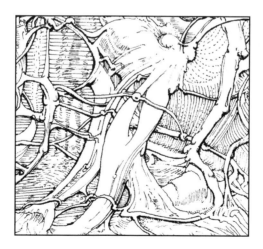

Fig. 29 Layers of fascia

This webbing can be seen as the interconnection of collagen fibers, or microscopically as the webbing of microfibrils with organized water between them. At both levels, the webbing is engaging and disengaging in response to pressure and movement, while creating a stable container for the body's functions.

All the different experiences in our life pulsate through the microfibrils/organized water matrix. They include the layers of wave motion that create our signature resonance, the layers of experience that shape and form our structure, and the layers of trauma that also shape and form our structure.

As we move through life our layers of experience are expressed in the quality and capacity of our bioelectric matrix. This layering of experience is mapped onto the crystalline organized water in the matrix. This memory helps the body respond to different movements and inputs from experience. When we have trauma in our lives, whether a car accident or life threatening situation, the memory in the matrix keeps the body aware of the signs and signals we need to respond to. When the trauma stays in the foreground of the matrix, it can diminish the mobility and motility of the matrix. When I work with trauma in clients, I am careful to engage with the whole, dynamic matrix in order to enhance an integrated experience.

WHAT CREATES THE LAYERS IN THE FASCIAL FIELD?

Esoteric as this may sound, the fascial field's layers are created by the wave motions of experience and function in the body. The different resonances that pulsate through the microfibril/organized water matrix are wave patterns that begin with the primitive streak. This first impulse creates the midline and begins the process of layering wave motion into the field. As the embryo develops, a heartbeat waves in the matrix field, as well as a cranial rhythm, long and mid tide rhythms, and other external and internal inputs. This layering of wave patterns creates an overall signature wave.

The fascial field layers are highly dynamic, holding the layers of experience and conducting them through the bioelectric matrix. The resonance of the field can be coherent and interconnected; alternatively, there can be interference in the field due to inertial patterns and isolated areas, which disperse and disconnect the resonance.

EXPLORATION 23: FINDING THE LAYERS WITHIN THE FIELD

Find a comfortable place to lie down and settle into your body. Let your awareness soften into the subtle vibrations in the matrix layers. Feel the subtle back and forth, ebb and flow of vibration in the organized water matrix.

Focus on the pulsations from the heart and feel how they move through the matrix in the thorax. Focus on the longer pulsation of the breath and feel how it moves out through the arms and legs. Focus on the pulsations of the cranial rhythm and feel how it rotates and spirals through the head and down the spine.

Now let your focus go to the whole matrix and feel your signature resonance as it ripples through the layers of your matrix. Move with those ripples through the fascia, letting the body engage all the layers of fascia, pulsating and rippling, toes to fingertips. Hold your awareness to the sensations of pulsation, then let them move you. When you feel a pause, soften into the subtle vibration again and witness its ebb and flow. Let it move you.

Come back to stillness and notice how you are sensing your body differently.

THE FASCIAL LAYERS AS A WEBBING

Because of the dynamic interconnectedness between layers of fascia, both fractally and within the space of the body, it is sometimes hard to distinguish between them. The fascia is like a webbing that is interconnected between functional spaces of different sizes. This webbing can be more horizontal, as in the diaphragm and pelvis, or more vertical, as around long muscles and bones. Science likes to differentiate and separate structures and name layers in the fascia, but they are so interconnected that they essentially cannot be separated.

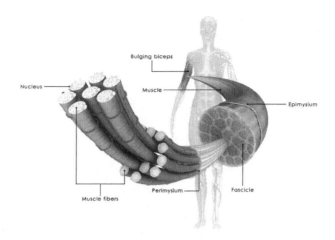

Fig. 30 Interconnected layers of fascia

We can palpate, contact and experience different levels of our matrix as our other tissues function, contract and expand. As you will see, when we pull and stretch any part of the webbing, the whole matrix responds.

THE MICROFIBRIL/ORGANIZED WATER LAYERS AS A CRYSTAL-LINE BIOELECTRIC MATRIX

The microscopic layers of microfibrils connect by organizing coherent water between them. These microfibril/organized water connections are arranged in different ways to give strength, flexibility and mutability to the fascia. Where strength and stability are needed, the microfibril/organized water matrix is layered in a multi-directional mapping. Such complexity of fibers holds and stabilizes, as well as shifts contact points to balance the tensions of movement. When the microfibril/organized water matrix is layered longitudinally, it supports our movements in gravity.

When the microfibrils build the fascial matrix, holding organized water for conductive pathways, they form a tetrahedron shape that gives greater connection, stability and flexibility. The microfibrils shift these tetrahedron shapes as a response to pressures and tensions, change in relationship to gravity, and movement. This shape is seen in all biotensegrity structures, including crystals (see Chapter 12).

When microfibrils shift and change their tetrahedral relationships as we move, changes ripple through all of the matrix layers. When at rest, they return to their learned configurations. The memory of rest and activity in the matrix is held in the crystalline water between the microfibrils. When the microfibrils are arranged as a complex, dynamic tensegrity system, the conductive and ionic capacity of the fascial matrix creates a crystalline coherent memory map informing the matrix of its past.

COMPARTMENTALIZATION

As discussed, the layers of fascia are a webbing of interconnected collagen fibers that create an information highway for the differentiated tissue systems of the body. When a muscle contracts, causing pressure on the fascia surrounding it, the rest of the body is aware of this movement and responds through the shifting of microfibril tetrahedral connections to help us balance reciprocal tensions in muscles and respond to gravity. This is what gives us the ability to play complex piano concertos or fly through the air to dunk a basketball. The millions of minute shifts in the microfibril connections are remembered in the matrix and can repeat themselves effortlessly with complex movement.

When any part of the body—be it muscle, tendon, organ or vessel—begins to draw away from the matrix's interconnectedness through injury, trauma, emotional mirroring or repetitive movement, it pulls the microfibrils together around itself and reduces its connecting tetrahedral arrangements, reducing its ability to reconfigure its crystalline memory. This compartmentalization of an area isolates and separates it from the information exchange of the whole body. Such an area no longer "remembers" it past connections, no longer takes in new information, and does not respond to new changes in reciprocal tensions.

Over time, a compartmentalized area will compress and increase in density, reducing the fluid capacity and flow of nourishment into the area. It is thus important to re-enliven the matrix, building new organized water pathways, so that the system can remember its patterns from the past, creating an awareness of the cumulative experiences of the organism. Fortunately, we can integrate the trauma experiences into our cumulative memory, allowing the matrix to continue mapping new experiences.

EXPLORATION 24: RECONNECTING YOUR LAYERS OF FASCIA

Find a comfortable position lying down and settle into your body. Bring your awareness to each layer of fascia, starting under the skin. Finding superficial and deep fascia, glide it so you can feel its shape and form.

Now shift your awareness to the myofascia and focus on the matrix wrapping around muscle fibers, muscle bundles, muscles and muscle groups. Follow the matrix as it connects and surrounds tendons, ligaments and bones. Glide around a muscle, tendon and bone feeling the integrity, sponginess and individuation around the tissue.

Now shift your awareness to the visceral fascia, feeling the matrix in the torso cavity and around the organs. Feel how they are individuated and separate while connecting through the matrix to the whole.

Shift your awareness to the internal matrix around the spinal cord (the dural tube). Glide it back and forth by gently nodding the head forward and back.

Focus back through the layers of fascia, gliding them individually. As you glide one layer, begin to use a stronger glide and rotation to begin to feel the connections between layers.

Now let your body move in the same gliding and rotating motions, letting the body determine the direction. Keep slowing down the glide and let the body pause and wait for an impulse to move it. Continue to let go of moving with your muscles and let the matrix move you. Notice the movement in the matrix away from where you initiate glide.

Come back to stillness and notice the different sensations you feel.

INTERRELATIONSHIP VS. ISOLATION

There is a significant difference between a tissue being interconnected with the whole body and being isolated from the whole body. Among other problems, an isolated, compartmentalized area begins to create its own resonance, sending mixed signals to the matrix. The crystalline memory in the matrix shifts and the body becomes clumsy lacking in coordination. The matrix in the body can be felt as dense, sticky, undifferentiated, hot or cold and lacking conductive flow. If this area continues to be isolated, it deteriorates and creates space for disease and toxicity to grow. But when we move the fascial matrix through specific movements, or reconnect it through touch, we are shifting the body's vulnerability back to vitality.

When your bioelectric fascial matrix is interconnected and all of the tissues are interrelated through them, your body's vitality, potency and conductivity are strong and resilient. The interrelationship within the fascia layers is primary in keeping your body vital and whole, ready to respond to all the inputs from the internal and external environments, ready to perform complex, practiced activities seamlessly.

MOBILITY, MOTILITY AND MUTABILITY

With healthy, interconnected layers of fascia, the enlivened body has the full capacity for mobility, motility and mutability. With mobility, the structure has the ability to glide between tissues and allow for diverse range of motion. With motility, the field can vibrate through its microfibril/organized water pathways, informing all cells. And with mutability, the structure and field have the ability to adapt to input immediately, by changing form, shape and quality of vibration.

These three capacities determine your quality of health and overall well-being; they help protect the body from disease and other potentially harmful inputs, and they provide the body with maximum energy efficiency, nourishment and adaptability. These are the qualities of a vibrant state of living, connected to the internal and external worlds. By using the practices in this book you can revitalize your matrix and bring optimal health back into your daily life.

EXPLORATION 25: FINDING YOUR MOBILITY, MOTILITY AND MUTABILITY

Find a comfortable position lying down and settle into your body. Begin by gliding the surface matrix through the extremities, gently flexing and extending the foot or hand, feeling the mobility of the matrix.

Glide through to deeper levels, using rotation and spiraling. Notice how the matrix moves around the other tissues, without pulling or pushing. Let that movement settle.

Now let the resonant wave pattern of your body ripple out from the midline through the organized water between the microfibrils. Once it comes to the surface of your body, feel it moving back to the center. Bring awareness to this ebb and flow in the matrix. Notice the strength, depth and quality of the wave motion's motility (pulsation out from the midline). Feel the motility of the whole system. Let that movement settle.

Now let your fascial matrix initiate slow movements throughout its layers. Notice how the matrix changes as it glides and spirals, adapting to any shift in position and in relation to gravity. Notice the mutability of the tissue as it adapts and recalibrates itself. Come back to stillness and feel the effects of the mobility, motility and mutability of the matrix.

LAYERING EFFECTS:

- Interconnectedness of tissues
- Differentiation of tissue
- Maintaining balanced reciprocal tension
- Conductivity of the matrix
- Information exchange
- Mobility
- Motility
- Mutability

INERTIAL PATTERNS AND LAYERING

When fascial layering is impaired, the layering compresses and increases in density, reducing complexity in the microfibril/organized water matrix. The collagen fibers bind together, over-stabilizing and reducing the area's range of movement. The bioelectric matrix's conductive capacity is reduced as the alignment and interconnectedness between microfibrils is broken, diminishing the exchange of information through the layer. This disconnection creates an inertial pattern that can create its own conductive rhythm.

When a fascial layer is impaired through injury, overuse, dehydration, lack of movement or repetitive movement, it becomes isolated and pulls into itself. This isolation disconnects it from the whole, integrated matrix. Sometimes, the rest of the matrix adjusts to this isolated area by pulling away from it. You can feel this pull throughout the matrix. Sometimes the matrix is pulled toward the isolated area, bunching fascial layers toward a center point, pulling away from the healthy matrix surrounding it. This can be palpated as a hardened area with tension around it. Sometimes it is tender to touch and tender with movement.

All of the different ways a tissue might react to trauma, injury and emotional sensations in the body can become inertial patterns in the fascial matrix. The inertial pattern reduces nourishment and information flowing into the matrix. The surrounded muscle or organ loses contact or relationship to other organs and muscles of the body. Proprioception, coordination and ease of movement in the area become distorted and clumsy. We begin to withdraw from movement and activity due to instability and lack of balance. This cycle continues to degenerate our level of health and vitality unless we re-enliven our matrix.

EXPLORATION 26: FINDING INERTIAL PATTERNS THROUGH THE LAYERS

Find a comfortable position lying down and settle into your body. Scan your body and find a place where there is discomfort, pain or a lack of sensation.

Focus on this place in your body. Start at the surface and feel the superficial and deep matrix at this place. Gently glide that part of the matrix and notice if it moves freely or is bound to the tissue around it. Now create a deeper glide and notice where the myofascial and visceral layers of the matrix move and what layers do not.

Let your gliding movement guide you to the layer that is stuck. Focus on that layer and begin to initiate a gliding movement *through* the stuck area. As the stuck area begins to move with the other layers, initiate rotations and spirals out into the rest of the body. Move through the inertial patterned area, reintegrating it to the whole matrix.

Notice the wave pattern within the isolated area, and initiate a rippling from the whole matrix into the inertial patterned area. Now ripple back and forth through the area in multiple directions, integrating the inertial waves into the signature wave of your organism.

Repeat this in other areas of discomfort, or again in the same area. Notice the layer or layers that are dense, struck or have their own wave pattern.

Come back to stillness and notice the different layers of the matrix and how they have shifted.

EFFECT OF TOUCH ON LAYERING

When a layer of fascia is impaired and creates an inertial pattern, both touch and movement can open the area and reconnect the fascial matrix layer back into the bioelectric matrix of the whole body. Finding the specific layer that is the source of impairment is important. Using touch to find the layer of concern, we can then glide that specific area into the whole.

When palpating an inertial pattern, your hands will find a dense, sticky, undifferentiated area within the tissue. As you penetrate into the inertial pattern you may find that the isolated area pulls you through a line in the matrix. You can glide that line back into relationship with the other layers.

Using pressure, glide, streaming or micro-figure eight movements, hands-on work can open isolated areas, liquefy the density, reduce the pull toward or away from the area, reconnect the area to the whole bioelectric matrix, and bring the reciprocal tension back into balance. The area begins to move and glide in response to shifts in the reciprocal tension and restores the body's wholeness.

EXPLORATION 27: TOUCHING THE LAYERS OF THE MATRIX

Start by settling your hands a foot apart upon the anterior thigh of your client. Let your upper hand gently pull up toward the hip, creating a tautness in the surface matrix. Now glide the matrix toward the tautness. Glide without moving across the skin, feeling the surface layer of fascia move. Notice the quality of movement and the fluidity of the glide.

Move back and forth, creating tautness with one hand before gliding the matrix. Notice the increase in glide and fluidity.

Now let your hand pull a tautness more deeply, letting your hand pull at a 30º angle, not moving across the skin. Penetrate the surface until you have contacted the matrix surrounding the quadriceps. Feel the thin layer of matrix in your hand. Glide this layer back and forth and in multi-directions. Notice how the glide is shorter and the quality of movement different.

Continue to deepen your touch until you contact deeper myofascial and the periosteum of the bone. Glide this thin layer of fascia. Notice how the glide is minimal at this level.

Now work back through the layers, lightening your touch to find the different layers. End by gliding the surface matrix in multiple directions. Take your hands off the thigh and repeat on other leg.

Once you have completed this, rest your hands on the thigh and let the matrix glide your hands in linear and spiral movements. Bring your hands out slowly, letting the matrix come to rest.

CASE IN POINT: INTRINSIC AND EXTRINSIC MATRIX DISCONNECT

When working with the layering nature of the structural matrix, one common disconnection is between the extrinsic (surface) and intrinsic (deeper) matrix. The surface fascia may respond to the constant external inputs by compressing and stiffening. This can be presented in the client as restricted and rigid posture or behavior. On the other hand, the surface fascia may be loose and fluid while the intrinsic fascia around the deeper muscles and viscera may be compressed, lacking the fluidity needed to slide and glide.

With either of these configurations, the bioelectric matrix will be disconnected and the information from the matrix near the skin will not resonate with the deeper information in the intrinsic matrix. This disconnect can be seen in the body's overall shape. In addition, the client may talk about not being comfortable in her skin, or perhaps say that she has a sense that she is two different organisms. Other telltale signs include specific sensations, a narrow range of motion, and frequent injuries.

Rachel came into my practice with multiple tender "trigger points" on the surface of her body. She stayed active, walking and going to the gym, but she found she was unable to increase her strength and energy levels. She was interested in finding new ways to address her limited life.

Rachel lay down on my table face up. I gave her a moment to settle in. When I put an impulse into Rachel's system at the feet, her surface matrix resisted and sent the impulse back into my hands. When I changed my direction of impulse towards the periosteum of the bone, it moved up the body easily without much depth. I began to work on the superficial layer of the surface matrix, sliding and gliding, using the flexion and extension of the foot to extend the glide. Once the surface fascial matrix began to move, I worked the deeper layer in the surface fascia to open and hydrate the surface layer. Then I continued to glide it laterally to medially, and I followed its spiraling up the leg. I used figure eight micro-movements at the ankle and knee, and I felt the glide of the surface fascia in the leg increasing. Next, I moved into the deeper layers and used the slide and glide to reconnect the surface to the deeper layers. Following the matrix movement through the legs, I found the layers reconnecting, and I felt a buoyant sponginess throughout the legs. I continued this up the hips, torso and arms, going from superficial to deep and back. I finished with gliding the dural tube and integrating the three layers in the structure.

The layers of matrix slowly returned to normal fluidity as Rachel and I continued working together. At each new session she started with a greater integration in her matrix, so I integrated superficial to deep, as well as working to integrate the field and restore the microfibril/organized water matrix through the layers. She found a new sense of vitality and was able to gain more strength in her muscles.

Another client, Rosanne, came in looking loose and relaxed, though she had recently strained her right shoulder, left hamstring and right Achilles in different episodes. These strains had compounded into pain when walking and an inability to exercise without significant discomfort. Rosanne was also concerned that she was feeling weaker day by day, and other symptoms included difficultly with digestion and assimilating food.

Rosanne lay down on the table, exhaling to relax. When I put an impulse into Rosanne's matrix, the surface layer of the matrix was loose and relaxed. But as I shifted the impulse to move into the matrix's deeper layers, I felt significant compression, a lack of conduction, and no glide between the layers. I began to feel for areas with the more density, and I worked at opening them by gliding the areas around them and bringing them back into connection. As the inertial areas I discovered began to reintegrate into the whole matrix, I glided the deeper fascial matrix up into the superficial fascial matrix, shifting the compressed and tensile relationship between the two. I worked up Rosanne's entire body, focusing on the denser areas, gliding and reintegrating them into the whole matrix. I finished by gliding the extremities and torso, superficial to deep, following the spiral movements of recalibration. I continued to work with Rosanne of the following months, concentrating specifically on areas of strain along with the fascial matrix of the viscera and torso. Many of her symptoms were soon relieved, and she began to feel more integrated, able to exercise and enjoy the daily activities of life.

CHAPTER 7
SUSPENSION/BUOYANCY

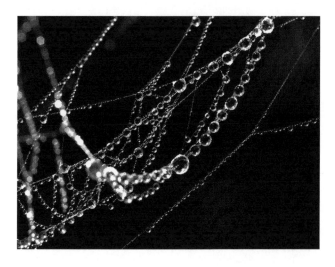

The air we breathe and move through is full of unseen particles that include fine particles of dust, pollution, microorganisms, moisture, oxygen, nitrogen, carbon dioxide and other chemical compounds, many of which may be classified as pollutants. These particles move through space, land on surfaces and move into living organisms to be used, exchanged or discharged. These unseen particles move through the air by wind patterns, rain patterns and ionic attractions. Sometimes they are pulled together by forces of attraction, while at other times they are pushed apart by forces of repulsion. The highly charged air creates a container where the particles within it are dispersed, shifting with molecular attraction, repulsion and movement. Moisture in the air is dispersed in the same way, creating mist and fog. Particles and moisture are differentiated within the space, available to connect with the Earth and its biosphere.

Like the air, the fluid ground substance in the fascia creates a medium for charged particles to disperse within it, which allows these particles to be available for the body to use. The highly charged fascia also allows organs and tissues to function without being pulled and tugged by the forces of attraction and repulsion, differentiating them and giving them access to molecules they may need.

This sort of suspension, whether in the air we breathe or the fascia we inhabit, allows the air particles or the body's functioning parts to be separate yet able to connect to the whole. The dynamic tension that exists between charged particles creates a container for other systems to function individually while still be connected to the whole. Thus these systems can stay contained to function efficiently instead of dissolving into the push and pull of dynamic forces surrounding it.

WHAT IS SUSPENSION?

Suspension is when a container is interconnected enough to allow the weight of its contents to disperse within the space of that container. In our body, this quality allows charged particles and nutrients to be suspended (or float) within fluid mediums instead of being pushed and pulled by the myriad forces around them.

There are three components that create suspension. First, the container provides the space for suspension to occur. Second, the fluid in that container is connected enough to allow particles within it to float without touching or reacting to each other. And third, the particles dispersed within the fluid are available when a force overcomes the suspension and moves the particle where it is needed.

WHAT CREATES SUSPENSION IN THE FASCIAL STRUCTURE?

The fascial structure creates suspension both in the macrocosm of the body and in the microcosm of the connective tissue. Put another way, the fascia is the container that allows the fluid and particles of each tissue system to be suspended within it. In the macrocosm of the body the fascia is able to suspend tissue systems so they can work independently of gravity and the push and pull from other systems, while creating a medium for exchange. When you palpate organs in the torso, you can feel how the lungs suspend in the pleura, how the heart suspends in the pericardium, and how the digestive tube suspends in the mesentery. These structures allow for spaciousness in a crowded container.

In the microcosm of the connective tissue structure, collagen fibers create the container, the ground substance creates the fluid medium, and the cells are suspended within the fluid of the structure. The microfibril/organized water matrix is also suspended in the fascia, giving it the independence and interdependence of a semiconducting pathway. Between the microfibrils, negative ions are suspended in the organized water, giving it the ability to conduct protons through it.

Suspension is an essential part of how we maintain a reciprocal tension within the fractal layers of our bodies. The drawing together of coherence and dispersal of suspension find balance in our fascial system, creating a buoyant, spring-like quality. This reciprocal tension between forces give us space and stability to move through the world.

When this reciprocal tension is impaired, and one force overrides another, our body uses muscle power to resist the pressures of gravity. When the matrix densifies and compresses, the suspension of the separate parts is lost. This impairs the flow of nutrients and toxins through the body, the flow of information in the organized water, and the overall flow of movement within the fascial matrix.

WHAT CREATES SUSPENSION IN THE FASCIAL FIELD?

The fascial field is created from ionic relationships within the microfibril/organized water matrix and its fluid medium. Within the organized water between microfibrils, negative ions align on the surface of the microfibrils and the positive ions pump through the water. This creates suspension in the organized water, so it can act like a semiconductor of wave motion and vibration.

When two particles of the same ionic charge come close together in the fluid matrix, they repulse each other, moving or suspending away from each other. When two particles of the opposite charge come close together, they pull together, suspending them away from the other particles of opposite charge in the medium. This push and pull balances to create suspension in the matrix, allowing for a greater movement of particles through the structure.

SUSPENSION IN THE BODY

The fascial webbing creates suspension for the various tissues it surrounds. It provides an interconnected container that allows the weight of the organ systems to disperse equally in the space it provides. This gives the tissue systems the capacity to function without having to constantly respond to outside forces. This container of fascia continually informs the tissue systems about the internal and external changes in the body while also providing space for them to function.

SUSPENSION IN THE FASCIAL STRUCTURE

The collagen fibers within the fascial structure create an interconnected container, allowing + and - ions and various cells to be suspended in the fluid medium of the ground substance. This allows the various cells to be available throughout the ground substance and fascia webbing, and it allows the charged particles to attract and repulse on another, moving, shifting and spiraling within the fluid medium. The ends of the collagen fibers also have + and – charges, giving them the ability to spiral and shift in response to movement and pressure.

The microfibril/organized water matrix organizes its + and – ions to allow for conduction through the organized water. The suspension the matrix creates allows for quick movement of protons and photons. You can also see this suspension inside cells.

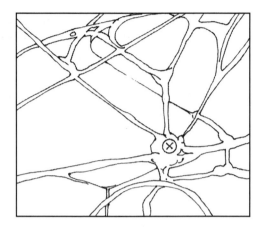

Fig. 31 Microfibrils of Fascia

SUSPENSION WITHIN CELLS

With the fractal nature of the universe, and the fractal nature of the body, we can see the same suspended nature on the micro-level of the cells themselves. The cell membrane is the container, essentially an interconnected, semipermeable medium of exchange. The cytoskeleton within the container creates the interconnectedness of the intercellular fluid. And the cell bodies are suspended within the cytoskeleton and fluid medium.

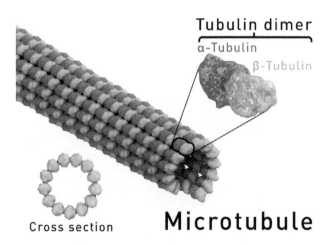

Fig. 32 Cytoskeleton of the Cell

106

You can see the fractal nature (see chapter 11) of the body when you compare the cells structure and the body's fascial structure, The structures of the cell include the cell membrane, cytoskeleton, fluid and cells bodies. These are self-similar to the collagen fibers, ground substance and cells within the fascial structure. This fractal nature connects the macro- and micro-levels of the body, mirroring each other in activity and response.

This suspended structure creates a dynamic, moving, changing medium where push and pull between ions allows the system to move protons and photons within its waters. This balanced tension allows the body to function efficiently without friction and resistance to change in movement. We call this balance between the charged particles the balanced reciprocal tension in the system.

EXPLORATION 28: FINDING SUSPENSION IN THE BODY

Find a comfortable position lying down on your back and settle into your body. Bring your awareness to your arm. Imagine that spaces inside the arm are being filled with air and extending outward in all directions. Feel the suspension and the lightness of the arm. Lift it up as if it is floating in space, as if it is lighter than air.

Repeat this process to create space and suspension in your other arm, torso, hips and legs. Let the suspension draw the areas up off the floor, floating in space. Feel the buoyant support from the air.

Now let your full body move from that suspended place, letting your legs move in arcs in the air. Let your body experience the suspension as a contrast to the weight of gravity. Use your breath to increase the suspension in the matrix, then glide the matrix from this buoyant place.

Come back to stillness and notice the sensations in the body.

Stand up, walk, move and spiral as you feel the buoyancy of the body and the support of gravity.

SUSPENSION AND COHERENCE

The charged particles in the fascial matrix create the dynamic between suspension (pulling apart) and coherence (pulling together). These charged particles are found at the ends of the microfibrils, as well as between them. This charged dynamic between the microfibrils in the organized water conducts protons through the center of the microfibril connections while the electrons line the inner surface. Thus the microfibril/organized water matrix has semiconductor qualities (like a high-speed information highway) and uses the balance of suspension and coherence to create a coherent domain. This ionic organization is stable enough to conduct information through its channels, but unstable enough to allow for shifts and changes in the microfibril connections. This shape-changing in the microfibrils gives us the capacity to interact easily with our environment and glide between both suspension and coherence. We can move fascially by gliding out through suspension and spiraling with coherence, or we can move muscularly through contraction and stretch.

BALANCED RECIPROCAL TENSION

Balanced reciprocal tension is created in the fascia through the attractive and repulsive forces of the charged particles of the microfibril/organized water matrix. The tension from these opposing forces engenders space and relationship to all the tissues of the organism and keeps them from collapsing or compressing in response to pressures and tensions from the internal and external environment.

In order to create stability in the continually changing matrix, the forces of suspension and coherence create an overall balanced reciprocal tension while they shift and change. They are continually recreating this balance with each conductive input. When the body glides with the rebalancing reciprocal tension, it expresses vitality, buoyancy, potency and enlivenment.

EXPLORATION 29: FINDING YOUR BALANCED RECIPROCAL TENSION

Find a comfortable position on your back with your arms and legs spread out from the torso. Settle into your body. Feel the tensions, holding patterns and push/pull within the body.

Place one arm above your head and gently glide the matrix from arm to leg and back, creating tautness by pulling the arm, then the leg, back and forth. Repeat on the other side of your body. Notice the reciprocal tension between the two sides.

Next, place one arm out to the side. Glide the matrix from one arm and opposite leg, creating tautness in one extremity and move the opposite one back and forth. Notice the reciprocal tension between the arm and opposite leg.

Now let the body initiate movement and notice the suspension and the coherence that shifts as the body moves. Use rotation and spiral movement to feel the complex reciprocal tension that shifts in the microfibril/organized water matrix. Come back to stillness and notice a different felt sense around your internal matrix.

BUOYANCY OR COMPRESSION

When your balanced reciprocal tension is active throughout the matrix, you can sense a buoyancy or lightness that gives you the ability to move and flow through the effects of gravity. When you feel this light and buoyant quality, the suspended nature within the fascia is transferred to your quality of movement and your relationship to the external world. You have probably known someone who moves effortlessly through life, with a positive, open, always curious attitude. Someone who seems so at ease wherever they are. This is the external expression of a balanced reciprocal tension, where the push and pull, pain and dis-ease of life are absent.

When the balanced reciprocal tension is impaired, whether in one area or many, those areas in the fascial matrix become compressed and reduce their ability to suspend. This compression brings a feeling of heaviness to the area and limits its range of motion and movement capacity. You may feel you are being pushed and pulled through life, instead of gliding through your day to day reality.

When such compression is present, it creates less space, less exchange and less relationship. This affects the fascia's ability to create space for the organ systems it surrounds, and it also affects the ability of that organ system to function.

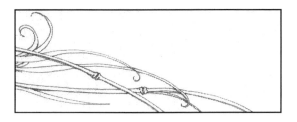

Fig. 33 Forming Buoyant Matrix

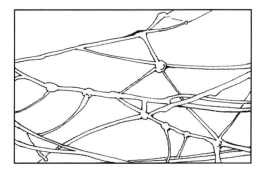

Fig. 34 Suspended Matrix

EFFECTS OF SUSPENSION

- Creates buoyancy and lightness
- Creates space for electron and proton exchange
- Creates a buffer to gravity
- Creates a conductive pathway
- Creates an interconnected container
- Creates movement with ease
- Creates vitality and potency
- Enlivens the system
- Contributes to the balanced reciprocal tension

EXPLORATION 30: SUSPENDING THE PSOAS

Stand with one hand on a wall or chair for support. Begin by imagining space expanding through your torso and up your neck and head. Lift your head upward slightly. Let your pelvis open out to the side, expanding.

Place your outside leg behind you and raise the same arm. Feel the suspension in the psoas muscle between the middle of the abdomen and the inner upper thigh. Move the leg back to create tautness in the area and raise your arm, gliding the matrix back and forth from the leg, through the torso, and up the arm. Feel the psoas suspending and supporting. Repeat other side.

Come back to standing and notice the sensation in your abdomen. Walk holding that suspension in your psoas. Notice any changes in your gate.

INERTIAL PATTERNS IN SUSPENSION

When our bodies create inertial patterns around injury, trauma, overuse and repetitive movement, suspension in that area is reduced. The charged particles begin to bind together and the ionic organized water is dispersed. This binding and dispersing creates dehydration, compression and density, reducing conductivity in the fascial matrix.

In cases like this, your body can become heavy, and its takes more energy for you to move. Your body resists the pull of gravity and you feel tension, pain and discomfort around the inertial pattern. Depending on where the inertial pattern is, your organs or muscles will function poorly and other symptoms around that area can arise.

Your inertial pattern may also create its own suspension, potentially putting pressure on the surrounding tissues. Or it may create its own conductive flow, pushing and pulling away from the surrounding tissue. All communication is reduced, and separate information may reinforce the binding in the area.

Through movement and touch, you can gently open and release the binding and bring the inertial pattern back into the conductive flow. When you release the binding you create more space inside the fascial matrix. The water reorganizes between the microfibrils, complexifying their connections and rebuilding your bioelectric pathway. These new conductive pathways reconnect into your body's flowing matrix, and the inertial pattern is cleared.

EXPLORATION 31: SUSPENDING YOUR INERTIAL PATTERNS

Find a comfortable positions lying down and settle into your body. Scan your body, noticing places of discomfort, disconnect and compression. Bring your awareness to one of these inertial patterns.

Begin by noticing the size, shape and sensation in the area. Notice the edges and depth of the area.

Begin to imagine the space outside and around the inertial pattern area expanding. Notice how the area inside of the inertial pattern responds. Feel its resistance.

Now imagine space expanding from the center of the inertial patterns outward in multiple directions. Keep expanding through the area and into the balanced area around it.

Now gently glide through the area in all directions. Feel how the suspension allows more layers of the matrix to glide with you.

Find other inertial patterns and repeat. Finish by letting the body move its internal matrix and integrate. Come to stillness and notice any changes in the body.

EFFECTS OF TOUCH ON SUSPENSION

When we use hands-on therapy to address the suspended nature of the fascia, we begin by creating more space for the tissues by spreading the matrix, maximizing suspension. This allows all of the tissues to have more differentiation and ability to function efficiently. This gives the fascia the ability to be the buffer as well as the information receiver for the body.

By gliding the fascia in all directions we reconnect it to the whole matrix and increase its conductive flow of information. The bioelectric matrix is able to shift from suspension to coherence easily when there are no blocked areas in its way. When the fascia is reconnected it restores the balanced reciprocal tension within the dance of this moving, changing medium. This increases vitality, potency and adaptability, nourishing and enlivening the whole body.

EXPLORATION 32: TOUCHING SUSPENSION IN THE FASCIA

Sit down facing your partner with you r hands on your thighs, palms up. First, focus on your hands and imagine your microfibril/organized water matrix inside them. Extend your fingers outward slightly and feel the matrix suspend and shift as you do. Now turn your hands over and place your palms on your partner's forearms, Make contact with the microfibril/organized water matrix in your partners forearms. Feel the pull into contact and then imagine your hands are pulling you partner's microfibril/organized water matrix away from their body, creating space in all directions. Feel the suspension that comes into the area you are touching.

Once you have felt the suspension in your partners forearms, slowly and gently glide their matrix in all directions. Notice where the glide gets stuck in the arm and reposition your hands to surround that area. Reconnect to the matrix and create space within it.

Continue to suspend and glide, gliding at different angles to include deeper layers of fascia. Let the tissue guide you to different areas of compression.

When you come to a pause, gently disengage your matrix from your partner's and lift off your hands.

Let your partner initiate glide in their fascial matrix. Ask your partner to describe their experience.

CASE IN POINT: HYPEREXTENSION AND COMPRESSION IN THE MATRIX

The compressive effects of gravity can be seen in the aging body as changes in height, collapse in the chest, and deterioration in hips and knees. Most of our repetitive movements also create compression in areas of overuse and draw the fascial matrix together. However, in some cases the body creates too much suspension and is unable to continually engage the shifting and changing of the fascial matrix. This suspended nature in the fascia can be seen in hyperextended joints, a narrowing of the body's depth, and more conduction moving toward the skin than inside the microfibril/organized water matrix.

Shirley came for a session presenting with carpal tunnel syndrome, which was causing numbing in her hands, pain in her arms and shoulders, and an inability to work out without significant discomfort in many parts of her body, including the hips, lower back and legs. Shirley was a gentle, quiet woman who spent much of her time rescuing others who had "worse" problems than she did. She worked long hours at the computer, and she swam and walked for exercise.

When I first put an impulse into her system after she lay on my table and settled in, the impulse swiftly moved up the outside of the body, disappearing as it went through the knees, and stopping at the hips. I felt a lack of density and compression and felt a hyperextension in the fascia.

I began my treatment by compressing the superficial fascia in the legs, first pulling together the fascia, then gliding the compressed matrix. I continued this into the deeper layers and used figure eight micro-movements, gradually making them smaller in areas where conduction was low.

I continued up through the hip, gliding the inner and outer fascial layers around the ilium and using compression on the sacroiliac joint to integrate the fascial matrix back into the whole. I continued up the torso, gliding her back muscles while drawing the fascial matrix toward the midline.

Next I worked with Shirley's shoulders, arms and hands, gliding through the joints and emphasizing the movement into the joint. I spread the retinaculum at the wrist with both my hands, then drew the fascial matrix back into internal spaces between the tendons. I continued to glide the arms, shifting to shorter glides to draw the fascial matrix back into a balanced reciprocal tension of compression and suspension.

I finished by gliding the dural tube, holding at areas of over-suspension and letting the fascial matrix reconnect and pull together. When I put an impulse in at the end of this session, the suspension was reduced and the compression was increased, enough to feel the intact fascial matrix of the whole body. The joints were conducting again and the tissue was more buoyant and spongy.

As we continued to work together, Shirley's over-suspended nature became a background issue and the inertial patterns that were hidden came to the surface. Her ligaments and tendons were more resistive and her muscles able to engage more fully. She was better able to exercise. Because of her long hours at the computer she eventually had surgery on her carpal tunnel issues, and by continuing to conduct the fascial matrix through that area, she has recovered fully.

CHAPTER 8
COHERENCE/EXCHANGE

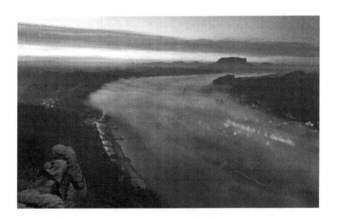

The fluid movement of water on our planet is a dynamic, coherent relationship of exchange. As the water in the seas, rivers and lakes evaporates into the atmosphere, the winds mix and move it around the globe. When that moisture precipitates as rain, snow or hail, it returns to the rivers, lakes and seas, changed by its relationship to the air and atmosphere. Some of the water gradually settles through the soil and rock, into the aquifers below the Earth. Here water is also changed by its relationship to earth particles, as it becomes our source of drinking water. Then, as we draw that water to the surface and into our bodies, we exhale and discharge this water back into the atmosphere returning it to the cycles of water on Earth.

This cycle of H_2O is consistent, interconnected and coherent. Within this coherent system, particles, chemicals and elements are exchanged, moving and shifting through the water medium. This coherent system is consistent and interconnected while also allowing individual parts within it to move and be used in different ways.

Like the fluid movement on the planet, the microfibril/organized water matrix of the fascia creates a coherent field of fluid for protons, photons and vibrations to move and be exchanged within. The organized water between the microfibrils, as well as the ionic push and pull between the microfibril structures, creates a coherent relationship that connects tissue systems to the whole while also allowing them to function independently. Just like water is an interconnecting medium on our plane—through its cycle between atmosphere, land and living organisms—the organized water inside and outside of our body's microfibrils of the fascia connects through it cycles of engaging and disengaging. And just like the individual particles of the Earth can move and relate to other particles through the coherent medium of water, the energetic rhythms of the body can move and relate to the individual tissues through the coherent domain between the microfibrils.

WHAT IS COHERENCE IN A LIVING SYSTEM?

Coherence in a living system is defined as the capacity to store incoming energy in a coherent form, closing the energy loop (so it doesn't drain away to entropy) into a regenerating life cycle. Coherent energy is created when this energy or wave ebbs and flows in an organized, consistent manner. A coherent domain holds the space for coherent activities to relate together and individually.

WHAT CREATES COHERENCE IN THE FASCIAL STRUCTURE?

Coherence—the ability to create order and consistency in a system—is found in the internal matrix of the human body. The microfibril/organized water matrix creates a coherent domain that can both store vibration and pulsate energy. This structure of ionic separation between protons and electrons, ordered in the water between the microfibril structures, brings the body to life.

This web-like, microfibril structure is also a coherent medium formed by molecular bonds (peptides) with + or - ions at their ends. This gives the microfibrils the ability to connect and disconnect as a response to movement as we change our relationship to gravity. These interconnected structures of organized water and microfibrils create a unified and ordered field in the body. These structures have the ability to conduct wavelike motions consistently and instantaneously to all parts, creating an energetic loop in the body. This is what we call the organized field of relationship in the body.

EXPLORATION 33: FEELING COHERENCE IN THE MATRIX

Find a comfortable position lying down and settle into your body. Bring your awareness to your internal matrix, following it from the superficial sleeve to the deepest level surrounding the spinal cord.

Breathing in, notice the expanding of the matrix and the coherence of the system as it changes its connection points to include the movement of the ribcage. Breathing out, notice as the matrix comes back in, it maintains coherence, connection and buoyancy.

Glide your torso from the midline out to the left side and back. Notice how the coherence and connection is maintained as you glide one way. Repeat the glide out the right side and back. Let these movements be gentle, slow and small. Move from the inside of the body and not through space.

Now let your matrix initiate the glide and notice the stability of coherence in the matrix as it shifts and changes. Keep relaxing your muscles and let your matrix glide and move you.

Return to stillness and focus on the coherence, integration and interconnectedness of the matrix.

WHAT CREATES COHERENCE IN THE FASCIAL FIELD?

Coherence in the fascial field is created by the unified, interconnected liquid crystalline matrix (see chapter 10). This energetic matrix of memory stores and circulates all the energetic relationships of the body through its webbing. The ionic, bioelectric makeup of the matrix field allows it to be a field of relationship for the body as well as a field of information exchange.

The matrix field is coherent and unified, pulsating at the organism's individual signature wave throughout the microfibril/organized water matrix, containing and protecting the energetic field of the organism.

EXPLORATION 34: MOVING WITH OUR COHERENT FIELD

Standing in an open space, feel the stability and grounding in your feet and settle into your body. Notice the wholeness of your matrix. Imagine your skin can sense beyond your personal electromagnetic field and into the Earth's field. Feel the relationship between the field of your matrix and the external environment.

From your own internal field, slowly move your internal matrix. Notice the coherence in your own field, and how it shifts and changes to the movement and the external environment's field. Let your matrix initiate your movement and glide through the external environment, feeling both the coherent field inside of you and the coherent field outside of you. Feel how they interact and how they glide around each other.

Come back to stillness and notice your coherent field and the external environment's field. Notice how they support each other in gravity.

COHERENCE IN THE MICROFIBRIL/ORGANIZED WATER MATRIX

Coherence in the microfibril/organized water matrix is created through the ionic connections between the microfibril amino acid chains and the organized water between them. Microfibrils are built from tropocollagen molecules in threes, spiraling into fibers. This protein building block arranges its atoms so hydrogen atoms make up the internal and external surfaces of the fiber. This draws the water molecules into a coherent arrangement between them. A conductive pathway is formed. This set-up is coherent but not permanent, allowing the microfibril amino acid chains the flexibility to shift, rotate, spiral and extend, while still maintaining its information highway.

Bruce Lipton, Ph.D.: "Most amino acids have positive or negative charges, which act like magnets… a protein's flexible back bone spontaneously folds into a preferred shape when its amino acid subunits rotate and flex their bonds to balance the forces generated by their positive and negative charges."

–From *The Biology of Belief*, Hay House, pg. 24.

FIELD OF RELATIONSHIP

The coherent ability of the microfibril/organized water matrix creates a field of relationship between our structure and field. Our field of relationship creates a rapid bioelectric field of communication, much faster than the nervous system. It is considered a quantum-level bioelectric field of action, and it behaves like a semiconductor, relaying the shifts and changes in our bodies instantaneously to all the cells in our body. This is what gives our body the ability to perform complex movements like typing on a computer, throwing a ball or playing an instrument. We become better at these complex skills with practice, because of the building of memory in the coherent field.

CRYSTAL MEMORY

Because of its coherent ability, the bioelectric field of the fascia creates some tension through the push and pull of ionic forces. These forces, when repeated in the same configuration, give the tissue "crystal memory." This is dynamically distributed within the structural network as a response to gravity and complex movement patterns, or statically distributed within inertial patterns of overuse, strain and repetitive movements.

Our matrix remembers both the developmental patterns of sitting, crawling and walking, as well as the trauma patterns from injuries, surgeries and emotional or physical abuse. This system continues to entrain memory patterns throughout our lives, reinforcing and shifting our repeating patterns. It is never too late to change and rearrange your crystal memory. You simply need to put new and diverse input into the matrix to complexify its repertoire.

STRETCHED   COMPRESSED

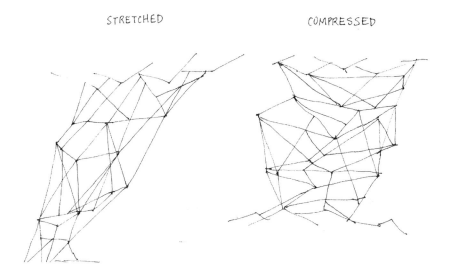

Fig. 35 Coherent matrix responding to forces

Mae-Wan Ho, Ph.D.: "As the collagens and bound water form a global network, there will be a certain degree of stability, or resistance to change, which constitutes memory; this memory may be further stabilized by cross-linking and other chemical modifications of the collagens. The network will retain memory of previous experiences, but it will have the capacity to register new experiences."

–From *The Rainbow and the Worm: The Physics of Organisms,* World Scientific, pg. 237.

EXPLORATION 35: MOVING WITHIN YOUR CRYSTAL MEMORY

Find a comfortable position lying on your back and settle into your body. Bring your awareness to your internal matrix of crystal memory. Let the internal matrix initiate a slow gliding movement. Focus your awareness on the movement pattern and notice how the matrix will repeat a movement pattern and then change the direction of the movement.

Let your body move until it is ready to be still. Relax into the stillness with open attention. Let the matrix initiate movement again and notice the movement patterns.

Come back to stillness and let your body relax fully. Stand up and walk slowly, noticing the matrix's patterns of walking.

COHERENCE VS. COHESION

Coherence is very different from *cohesion*. To repeat: coherence is an interconnected, organized relationship of pulling together, within which interconnected parts can change and shift to the internal and external demands of the system.

Cohesion, on the other hand, is the sticking together of a substance that binds and holds its contents, dissolving the individuality of the parts of the substance. In cohesion, the substance has no capacity to relate or exchange. Coherence creates a dynamic, open enlivened system, while cohesion creates a static, closed, inert system.

STABILITY AND MUTABILITY

The coherent bioelectric system is constantly exchanging information and wave motion through its webbing. Microfibrils are constantly changing connection points to respond to internal and external inputs. This mutability and adaptability happens continually and gives the body the dynamic, interconnected capacity to respond to the environment as a whole being.

The coherent bioelectric system creates stability through its balanced reciprocal tensions of ionic forces within the system. Because of the self-sufficiency of our matrix system and its ability to be stable and mutable at the same time, we can connect and disconnect to the external environment, exchanging information with it while still maintaining our unique individuality. Thus we have this capacity to connect to the external matrix of the planet without letting it overwhelm us.

EXPLORATION 36: CONNECTING THE INTERNAL AND EXTERNAL MATRIX

Stand and feel the support of the floor under your feet, as well as the coherence of your internal matrix. Bring your awareness to your internal matrix. Map your way through the layers of connection from the cell's matrix to the fascial matrix. Imagine their fibers are interconnected, pulsating information between them.

Now shift your awareness out to the inner and outer layers of your skin. Feel the coherence between the blood-side and air-side of your skin.

Imagine your microfibrils are reaching out to the surface of your skin. Imagine they are connecting to the matrix of the external environment. Let them connect and exchange information, giving contact and exchange.

Begin to move in that space, staying connected to the external matrix of the biosphere. Notice how the internal and external matrices move and dance with each other as you move. Come back to stillness. Disengage your microfibrils and let your internal matrix move, bringing your awareness back to your internal coherence. Notice your new felt sense of your internal and external worlds.

EFFECTS OF COHERENCE

- Creates an ordered, interconnected microfibril/organized water matrix
- Creates a medium for consistent exchange
- Unifies the liquid crystalline matrix
- Allows individual systems to function within an integrated whole
- Creates mutability and stability
- Creates a field of relationship
- Allows for crystalline memory within the
- changing, moving matrix

INERTIAL PATTERNS AND COHERENCE

When the bioelectric matrix is impaired due to stress, strain, injury, trauma, overuse or a narrow use of movement, the coherence in the area is reduced. As the collagen fibers begin to bind, crosslink and change chemically, coherence in the system is no longer able to thrive. Areas of inertial pattern become cohesive, essentially sticking together. The dynamic, moving, changing, mutable capacity of our matrix is restricted, creating a static, compressed, stagnant area. This inertial pattern becomes isolated and sometimes creates its own resonating matrix. This isolation creates further binding and deterioration of the fascial matrix, and it can isolate the tissues surrounding it.

With reduced coherence in such an area, we can no longer shift and change with pressure and tension, pulling on surrounding tissue and causing injury and strain. This also reduces our capacity to resonate wave patterns and rhythms through our bodies. This isolation and reduction of function reduces the dynamic, enlivened nature of the area, leading to deterioration and opening the area to disease and deconstruction. We are usually made aware of these areas when our sensory nervous system and proprioceptors relay the information to our central nervous system. Our brain processes this information and responds with sensations of pain, pull, resistance and disconnect.

EXPLORATION 37: FEELING THE CHANGE IN COHERENCE AROUND YOUR INERTIAL PATTERNS

Find a comfortable position lying down and settle into your body. Scan your body and find an area of discomfort, compression or disconnection. Bring your awareness to this area.

Begin by gliding the matrix around the inertial patterned area and notice how the coherence and connectivity changes as you start to glide into the area. Glide in multiple directions, slowly and gently, so you can feel the difference in smoothness of the glide and the amount of resistance in the inertial patterned area. Keep your glide small enough to stay within the isolated area.

Now focus inside the inertial pattern and do small figure eights within it. You can imagine making figure eights in the area, or you can use minute figure eight movements. Notice how the area softens and starts to change.

Gently glide from outside the area into its center again and imagine the microfibrils of the coherent matrix reconnecting to the microfibrils in the inertial pattern, building organized water between them. Glide through the inertial pattern to integrate it back into the whole matrix.

Come back to stillness. Notice the coherence in the area. Repeat in other areas of disconnection.

EFFECTS OF TOUCH ON COHERENCE

When bodywork practitioners use touch to contact the wave motion in the fascial matrix and feel the coherence in the system, we are connecting our own wave motion with our clients.

By letting the hands float into the dynamic fascial matrix, we can feel the quality and pace of the client's wave patterns. When we create an impulse with our own coherence, we can begin to shift the energy flow in the matrix.

We can enhance the energy flow or slow it down. We can use our own coherent impulse to open the inertial patterns in the system and reconnect them to the client's own coherence.

Touching the liquid crystalline matrix enhances the ionic exchange in the system, enhancing the healing capacity, potency and mutability of the fascia. By opening up inertial patterns we can reestablish the coherent nature of the system, enhancing the conductive and adaptive capacity of the body. By shifting and changing the crystal memory, we can reduce tensile contractive restrictions and bring more range of movement to the body. Reconnecting the fascial matrix and reestablishing the body to its interconnected coherence brings the body back into the dynamic, enlivened, vital potential that is innately present and possible at any time in our lives.

EXPLORATION 38: FEELING THE PULL OF COHERENCE

Take two attracting magnets and hold them between your fingers with their magnetic attraction facing each other. Bring them slowly towards each other until you can feel a slight resistance. Notice the change of sensation as they move close enough to create a pull. Continue to move them closer together, feeling the pull of connection. Notice the strength of the pull between them. This pull of positive to negative charges is part of what creates coherence in the microfibril/organized water matrix.

Next, put the magnets down and now find the magnetism in your hands. Rub your hands together for a minute or two, then hold your palms facing each other a foot apart. Slowly bring your palms together noticing when the energy between them.

Bring the palm of one hand down toward any place on your body and notice the coherence of connection as your microfibril/organized water matrix makes contact.

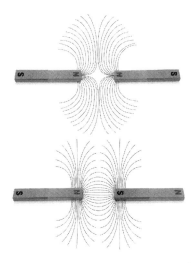

Fig. 36 Magnetic Forces

EXPLORATION 39: TOUCHING COHERENCE (WITH A PARTNER)

Start by focusing on your hands, bringing your awareness to the internal matrix in your palms. Imagine that your microfibril/organized water matrix is shifting its attention outward from the palms.

Next, bring your palms slowly into contact with your partner's thigh, with your partner either sitting or standing. Feel the connection between your matrix and theirs. Feel the coherence in your partner melt into your own coherence. Keeping your hands still, focus on the sensations in your palms and fingertips, noticing the subtle, shimmering vibrations and the ebb and flow in your partner's leg. Let the coherence inform your hands of the push and pull, ebb and flow within your partner's matrix.

Now follow that coherent movement, gliding your matrix and your partner's together. Let your whole matrix move your partner's matrix. Notice how the two matrices are informing one other as they dance and move.

Bring your hands back to stillness and slowly remove them, disengaging from your partner's coherent matrix. Notice the change in the sensations in your hands, and glide your own matrix to feel any change in coherence.

CASE IN POINT: INTEGRATING LEFT AND RIGHT, BALANCING THE COHERENT BOUNDARY

Cathy came in to my office with moderate discomfort in her left shoulder, as well as some heaviness in her chest. She was very active and her body was strong and flexible, but she was feeling distressed by her discomfort.

When I put an impulse up her body through her feet, I noticed that her right side was fluid and loose, with little boundary or coherence. Her left side had two inertial fulcrums at the hip and shoulder, with the area between pulled in tensile resistance. Her left and right sides were disconnected.

I worked her right lower leg to see if I could bring some coherence to the whole leg, and I realized that I needed to connect the lower legs. After gliding and streaming one leg, then the other, and then both, I moved up to Cathy's hips and continued to connect the left and right sides of her matrix.

Next I returned to the right leg, flexing the foot and drawing the hip bone upward to glide the tissue and enhance the conductivity. By helping the matrix find its left/right relationship through the midline and bring coherence across the body, the matrix was also able to bring coherence back into the right side. This could be felt by the buoyancy and sponginess of the matrix through the leg and hip.

I moved to the left side and worked the two inertial fulcrums at the hip and shoulder. I used figure eight movements in the inner part of the ilium and glided the matrix from the inside to the outside of the hip and back. I opened the compressed area and let the matrix shift and reconnect between the two inertial fulcrums.

Working with the right shoulder, I glided the tissue across the chest to the humerus and around the scapula to the posterior ribs. I worked under the arm, streaming the matrix through the joint from the top of the shoulder to the ribs under the arm. In some places the glide was very small, and in other places the glide twisted around the joint from bottom to top. Using a glide in many directions, I found the places where the matrix was disconnected.

I finished in the neck, gliding and streaming through the surrounding muscles. Finding my midline, then finding Cathy's midline, I followed the pulsations at the base of the skull and through the cheek bones, keeping my focus on the midline.

In the end, I found that Cathy's left and right sides were reconnected and the coherence of the whole system was now strong and buoyant. There was a greater depth of pulsation and the sponginess of the matrix gave and released with ease. Cathy said she felt more integrated, energetic and realigned.

CHAPTER 9
BALANCED RECIPROCAL TENSION

Balanced Reciprocal Tension is the dynamic balance between opposing forces that creates a buoyant, open system in our internal matrix. The structure of the spiraled, water-filled microfibrils sets up a container for water to separate its positive ions from its negative ions, and balanced reciprocal tension within that water provides a conductive pathway. Coherence holds the energy circulating in the microfibril/organized water matrix, and suspension gives space for the energy to move. This balanced reciprocal tension of coherence and suspension enables the matrix to create a coherent domain of stability, and to allow for mobility within its connections.

In the structure of the fascia, the pulling together and apart from the charged protein collagen fibers creates a balanced tension throughout the webbing, giving space and protection to the tissues it surrounds. Our matrix sets up changing compression and tensile forces as it responds to our movements.

The fascial matrix fosters a dynamic, buoyant environment for the body to move through gravity and respond to the external electromagnetic field. The body's dynamic tension is constantly changing and adjusting, both to internal and external pressures. Gravity creates a downward force toward the Earth, and we neutralize this force with our dynamic balanced reciprocal tension. As we move and bend and extend, our dynamic tension shifts immediately so we can stay upright and move through space with the least amount of counterforce and energy output. This dynamic tension in our fascia influences our balance, righting and equilibrium mechanisms.

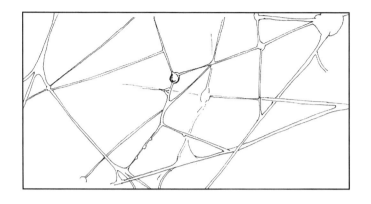

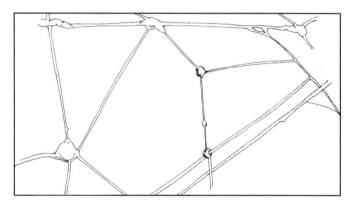

Fig. 37a and Fig. 37b Tensegrity Balancing

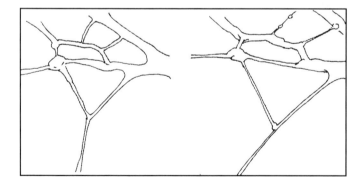

Fig. 38 Shifting matrix with pulling forces

POLARITY, COMPRESSION AND MULTIDIMENSIONAL TENSIONS

Our fascia creates a balanced reciprocal tension in order to reduce the impact of the pressure and tensions from our internal and external environments. The fascia responds to these inputs by shifting its microfibril/organized water arrangement to keep our bodies upright, stable and grounded.

These pressures can push and pull in different ways, asking our bodies to respond differently to each input. Some of the pressures can be seen as push or pull toward or away from our midline. Other pressures are compressing, pushing towards the midline of our body. These forces can come from the outside or from the tight muscles inside us. They can be one directional or multidirectional.

Some pressures can come from polar forces pulling at right angles to the midline. These forces come from our left or right hand dominance, imbalances in the left or right sides of our body, or shearing forces along the spine. These pressures create binding around or sideways shifting of the spine, reducing the shock absorbing capacity that our discs provide.

Other pressures are multidimensional, spreading out from our midline or from a center point, pulling away ionic attractions and reducing our body's coherence.

When these forces are dispersed and neutralized through the shifting microfibril/organized water matrix, the forces that create pressure on our organism have little influence on the functioning and integrity of our individual tissue systems. As the microfibrils shift and change their connections, the webbing remains intact and stable while our body disperses the forces upon it. When these forces pull and push the microfibrils into fixed and bonded configurations, inertial patterns are created in our fascial system.

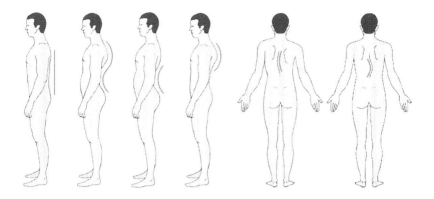

Fig. 39 Postural Alignments

EXPLORATION 40: FINDING THE DIRECTIONS OF TENSION IN THE BODY

Find a comfortable place to lie down and settle into your body. Scan your body and notice any differences you find… left and right, top and bottom, front and back. Notice where your body doesn't touch the surface you are lying on. Notice where there is tension and resistance. Notice the curve of your spine.

Begin gliding your matrix by gently flexing and extending your foot. Feel a gentle pull gliding up through your leg to the hip. Notice where there is resistance to your glide. Notice where there is no sensation of glide.

Bring your awareness to the area of resistance. Relax around that resistance and let your matrix begin to move. Follow the movement pattern and direction of tension that your matrix glides along.

If your fascia resists movement, initiate a glide around the area and notice the difference in the patterns inside and outside of the resistance. Repeat with your other side.

Pull your glide up into the torso, arms, neck and head by extending through your upper body. Notice where there is tension as you glide, where the movement pattern of your matrix changes.

Come back to stillness and scan the body again, noticing the differences.

MIDLINE AS NEUTRAL

Our body understands its relationship to gravity by using the midline (the mesodermic center) as its guide. Our midline was first formed before birth by the primitive streak, creating center and our first wave pattern. Our body uses midline throughout our lives to access neutral, where we don't have to respond to forces of push and pull. When we bring focus to the midline, we are able to find the stillness that resides within the balanced reciprocal tension.

Charles Ridley: "By consciously holding the reference point of the midline we allow what has lost relationship to the organization of the whole to come back into coherence connection."

–From *Stillness: Biodynamic Cranial Practice and the Evolution of Consciousness*, **North Atlantic Books, pg. 59.**

LAYERS OF BALANCED TENSION

There are many layers of dynamic tension in the body that give us balance, potential energy and our space in the world. There is a surface tension in our bodies that gives protection and helps our skin relate to the external world. Our superficial fascia shapes this dynamic tension. Our muscular tension or tonus is shaped by our fascia's reciprocal tension. There is also the cranial membranous balanced tension that affects our deepest layer of fascia. All of these layers of push and pull influence the reciprocal tensions in the matrix.

When our fascia glides over other tissues, reconfiguring its microfibril relationships and referencing through our midline, our body can move towards a balanced reciprocal tension. But when these forces cause binding in our layers of fascia, our reciprocal tension looks for balance around inertial patterns. This changes our proprioception, balance and use of energy. Our potency and vitality are impaired.

EXPLORATION 41: GLIDING AROUND THE LAYERS OF TENSION

Find a comfortable place to lie down and settle into your body. Bring your awareness to your skin. Feel the sensations on the outside and inside surface of your skin. Then move your awareness to the superficial fascia under the skin and gently glide it in multiple directions by moving your hands and then your feet. Notice the areas of push and pull, resistance and isolation. Notice the areas where the glide is smooth and strong.

Allow your glide to feed into the middle layers of fascia by spreading or rotating your extremities, create a glide deeper and in multiple directions. Notice where the matrix glides smoothly, quickly, slowly or with stilted movement.

Initiate movement from your midline out to your skin surface in any direction. Notice the layers of matrix as you glide out and in. Change the direction of your glide and notice where there is resistance or where other tissues shift movement qualities.

Let your matrix initiate movement and notice how it glides around your layers of tension, gently bringing them back into coherence.

Come back to stillness and notice the different sensations in your layers of tissue.

COMPLEXITY OF THE MICROFIBRIL/ORGANIZED WATER MATRIX

As previously stated, the microfibril/organized water matrix is the hidden webbing that vibrates our enlivened body. The matrix's ability to shift with different tensions allows us to move effortlessly and adapt to our internal and external environments. Some of our microfibrils align with the vectors of repetitive movement patterns, strengthening and stabilizing. When our collagen fibers compress and bind together the result is over-stabilization, which in turn reduces the complexity of our microfibril connections. Without varied movement, the microfibril connections weaken and lessen, reducing our adaptability and versatility of movement.

By consciously varying our movement in different directions and rhythms, we complexify our microfibril connections, giving them mobility and variety of movement potential. With complex, tensegrity-like arrangements within our microfibrils, we can move in diverse ways, quickly adapting to out environment. This versatility supports and bolsters our abilities to play complex music, or to leap, roll and twirl as a dancer. It is also what enables us to multitask in our daily activities, such as gesturing while talking, or singing and laughing while driving.

By moving our fascia in diverse directions (or getting hands-on therapy to unwind our compressed fibers), we increase the complexity of our microfibril/organized water matrix, creating a felt sense of buoyancy, space, coherence and suspension. We enhance the vitality and potency of our organism and participate in an enlivened, dynamic experience of life. Our system stays ready to engage in complex tasks, utilizing its whole integrated self.

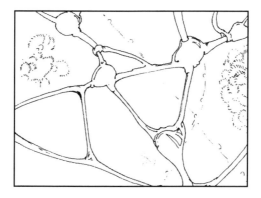

Fig. 40 Complex Matrix

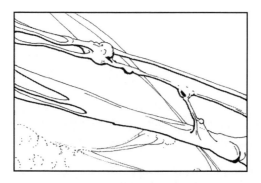

Fig. 41 One directional Matrix

EXPLORATION 42: COMPLEXIFYING OUR MICROFIBRIL CONNECTIONS

Find a comfortable place to lie down and settle into your body. Scan your body and notice the different sensations of density, resistance, fluidity, depth and integration.

Imagine you can explore the microscopic dimensions of your body. Let your awareness move through the fascial layers, finding the collagen fibers and then the microfibrils. Bring your imagination and awareness to the organized water between your microfibrils. Go to a specific area of your body and imagine you are swimming through the conductive fluid pathways. As you come to the intersections between the microfibrils, move from one pathway to another. Notice where there are a lot of intersections and where there are few.

Let go of the images you have used to find your matrix. Relax into your fascial webbing in your chosen area. Bring your awareness to the gentle movements within your matrix.

Let your matrix begin to move and glide in multiple directions in the area, while still keeping your awareness at the intersections of your microfibrils. Feel how they separate and reconnect at different points. Glide in directions where there is no intersection and feel your microfibril shift and connect in new ways. Repeat in other areas.

Finish by letting the matrix glide, integrating its new complexity.

EFFECTS OF BALANCED RECIPROCAL TENSION

- Creates a righting mechanism
- Creates integrated stability
- Can change from compression to suspension
- Creates surface tension for safety
- Creates space for organs to function
- Creates buoyancy
- Creates balance between gravity and midline

BALANCING RECIPROCAL TENSION

Your body's reciprocal tension is in a constant state of adjustment. This is because the body is in constant motion, whether from moving through space, autonomically regulating internal movement, tides and rhythms within the body, or resonant waves pulsing through the microfibril/organized water matrix. Your body never fully settles into a static state of balanced reciprocal tension. Nevertheless, because these changes happen immediately and around a complex, web-like structure, the fascial matrix remains stable and supportive, holding its spaciousness and alignment. The more you move in diverse ways, the more complex your microfibril connections are, the more you can move in small complex patterns, expressing yourself exquisitely as an artist, dancer, musician or athlete. In daily life, this complexity in your microfibril connections gives you greater capacity to respond quickly and effortlessly to the challenges of modern life, without reacting with fear or anxiety.

To create a moment of balanced tension in your body, you can pull up the slack within your fascia through a gentle pull on your matrix, until you feel a pause in internal movement. This stimulates your internal matrix to move, unwinding its fibers and complexifying its microfibrils. This helps to bring suspension and space back into your body, sustaining a web of tensegrity (see Exploration 43 below).

EXPLORATION 43: PULLING UP SLACK TO LET TISSUE UNWIND

Find a comfortable place to lie down and settle into your body. Let your spine, torso and extremities relax. Breathe and let your whole body relax with each exhale.

With your arms out to the sides and your legs hip distance apart, begin to gently pull away from the midline through your torso, first out to your hands, then out to your feet, then up through your head. Create a tautness from torso to extremity without pulling on your muscles, tendons and ligaments. Let your body relax into this tautness. Focus on your matrix and notice how it is moving, rippling, vibrating, heating and shifting in response to this tautness. Let your matrix unwind through this subtle internal movement.

When the unwinding settles down, gently pull back toward your midline, a creating tautness near the surface of your body. Let the tautness spread out on the surface. Feel it begin to move in different directions, unwinding your patterned matrix.

Come back to stillness and notice the change in your level of relaxation. Breathe and let your body reconnect, reintegrate and settle into its new matrix patterns.

WHEN FASCIAL RECIPROCAL TENSION IS IMPAIRED

When the fascia's ability to move into a balanced reciprocal tension is limited, your body becomes heavy, its movements stilted. This happens when you limit your movement patterns to sitting and walking. When you hold your body in one position, your fascia begins to stabilize in this position and in its relationship to gravity. It takes significantly more energy to move from this over-stabilized posture, and the body tends to push and pull, fighting with gravity. Collagen fibers become compressed and microfibrils simplify their configurations. Inertial patterns can develop, becoming fulcrums of tension and limitation.

When your body is bound by a sticky, over-compressed matrix, it is unable to function, communicate and respond internally. Movement pulls on nerves and tissues, creating pain and burning, while your matrix increases its binding, trying to create more stability. When this pattern continues, compression becomes isolation; blood flow and nerve flow are reduced, giving way to disease and allowing deterioration to increase inexorably. To restore balanced reciprocal tension, you can use touch and/or movement to glide and spread the matrix, increasing its ability to rearrange.

EXPLORATION 44: FEELING IMPAIRED RECIPROCAL TENSION

(see Chapter 23 for hands-on instruction)

Find a comfortable place to lie down and settle into your body. Scan your body and find an area of compression, discomfort or limited range of motion. Choose an area that you can reach with one of your hands. Bring your awareness to your matrix in this area.

Place your hand on the area and gently glide the superficial matrix. Don't move across your skin but pull up the slack and glide inside your skin. Feel the density, as well as the lack of buoyancy and sponginess.

Glide into the deeper matrix of the impaired area by pulling slightly more with your glide. Notice where the glide is more limited. With one hand, hold to the side of the impaired area where there is limitation of glide. Now glide your matrix in multiple directions with your other hand, gently moving away from your stationery hand. Shift the direction or placement of your hands to increase the depth, direction and length of the glide.

Let go of this area and let it glide on its own. Feel the changes in the impaired area.

Let your whole matrix glide to reintegrate the entire system. Come back to stillness and notice the sensations in the body.

EFFECTS OF TOUCH

The use of physical touch can be very powerful in balancing reciprocal tension in the body. When you use hands-on techniques to address impairments in the body's reciprocal tension, you pull up the slack in the fascial layers, giving the matrix a chance to unwind and the microfibrils a chance to complexify.

You listen and follow the fascial movements until you can move it in all directions, and you spread the fascial tissue to create space within over-compressed areas. You glide the fascial tissue to bring the collagen fibers into conductive relationship and help the microfibrils reconnect in new patterns. You hold the inertial patterns to let the fascia unwind itself and reconnect to the whole integrated matrix. You use impulse to stream through the conductive matrix, enlivening and restoring its capability for balanced reciprocal tension.

By using hands-on techniques, you can reduce compression, density and fulcruming around inertial patterns. You create space for the organs to function. You reconnect the bioelectric matrix. You open and reconnect inertial patterns, enhancing the coherence and integration of the whole.

EXPLORATION 45: HANDS-ON UNWINDING (WITH PARTNER)

Have your partner lie on her back on a massage table or bed, and give her time to settle into her body, relaxing with her breath. Have her scan her body and notice places of compression, discomfort or tension.

Begin by placing your hands around one of your partner's areas of discomfort. Let one hand create a tautness to the other hand, feeling the matrix begin to unwind.

Let your hands move with the movements of your partner's matrix and notice the directions that it wants to move back and forth. Let your partner's matrix move as long as it wants, following it or just witnessing it under your hands.

When your partner's matrix pauses, begin to initiate a gentle glide in the matrix between your hands. Shift directions, gently helping it move through resistance.

Move your hands to different areas. Start by creating a tautness — listening, following and then moving your partner's matrix in multiple directions, restoring its reciprocal tension.

Slowly and gently remove your hands from your partner. Ask her to describe her experience and the changes of sensation in the areas worked.

EXPLORATION 46: BALANCING RECIPROCAL TENSION (WITH ONE OR TWO PARTNERS)

Sit facing your partner with your legs crossed. Sit close enough so that you can hold your partner's arms at the elbows.

With a firm grip on your partner's arms, gently create some reciprocal tension between you. Feel the pull and resistance as you gently lean back, pouring your weight into your back space. Have your weight only pull at the arms until you feel tautness in your arms. Spread that tautness evenly through your torso and legs.

Release your pull and let your partner pull to tautness, spreading the pull evenly into their torso and legs. Have your partner release. Now have both of you pull to tautness, spreading the resistance evenly into your torsos and legs. Now let your bodies slowly begin to move, feeling the reciprocal tension shift and change in the matrix as you maintain your relationship to gravity and your partner's pull. Try to keep the same level of tautness as you move.

Come back to center and release your hold. Focus on your midline and let your matrix glide gently, restoring your reciprocal tension back to the midline.

With three people, sit with your legs crossed and creating a triangle.

Reach your arms out to the side to grasp the arms of your two partners, at or close to the elbow. Begin with one person creating tautness with both their arms, spreading it into their torso and legs. Let each person create tautness individually. Then have all three bring tautness to the triangle, spreading it evenly into your torsos and legs.

Begin to move slowly with an even and consistent amount of tautness, feeling the reciprocal tension shift and change as you move.

Come back to center and release your hold. Focus on your midlines and let your matrix glide gently, restoring your reciprocal tension back to the midline.

CHAPTER 10
LIQUID CRYSTALLINE MATRIX

The *liquid crystalline matrix* is the medium that creates the enlivened capacity of connective tissue. It is fractal in nature and can be traced through the intercellular matrix within the cell to the matrix of the fascia. Through the organizing of ions in the waters of the matrix and the coherent domain it maintains, the crystalline matrix maps its configurations, giving our bodies a memory of all our experiences.

Our liquid crystalline matrix is composed of a richly coherent organized matrix in which microfibrils build organized structures of water between them in biotensegrity forms of tetrahedrons (see Chapter 12). This liquid crystalline water conducts our wave patterns and ions through the matrix, allowing for the immediate exchange of information. Our microfibrils move and spiral as their ions dance, engaging and disengaging at multiple points when responding to push and pull, tension and pressure. This crystalline matrix conducts wave motions propelled by the internal processes of the body, as well as trapping and moving photons of light from the electromagnetic forces of the Earth.

The liquid crystalline matrix, through its bioelectric field, creates tension that responds to inputs of tensile and contractive forces. This, along with crosslinking and chemical modification of the collagen fibers, gives the tissue "crystal memory," which is dynamically distributed in the structural network. With all of the moving, changing and memory capacity, the amazing stability that is created through the balanced tension in the matrix gives the body the capacity for astonishing adapting, healing and performing in this complex world.

Charles Ridley: "...the whole bodily system is linked from the extracellular to intracellular by the connective tissue via specific microstructures that traverse cell membranes---all of which are suspended in a liquid crystal matrix."

–From *Stillness: Biodynamic Cranial Practice and the Evolution of Consciousness,* North Atlantic Books, pg. 181.

WATCHING THE MICROFIBRILS MOVE AND CHANGE

Jean-Claude Guimberteau, MD, is a pioneering French surgeon and medical researcher. In his work, Guimberteau has placed a high-powered microscope under the skin of a patient's forearm and watched the microfibrils move and change as the tissue is moved by the end of the microscope. His video is an amazing sight to watch: Living fascial tissue at the microscopic level and its dynamic dance of relationship. You can watch the water molecules move along between the microfibrils as the fibrils shift and change their relationship. You can watch the microfibrils extend to connect to another microfibril, or split into two fibrils to connect in a different way. When you add a push or pull to the fascia, the microfibrils begin to dance by joining and separating, pulling together and drawing apart. This dance continually responds to the wave motions and shifts in gravity, while the whole fascial webbing maintains a tensegrity of strength and stability. We are mostly tuned to the stability and solidness we feel in our bodies, but what would it be like to be tuned into the spiraling motion and pulsations that constantly move and change it?

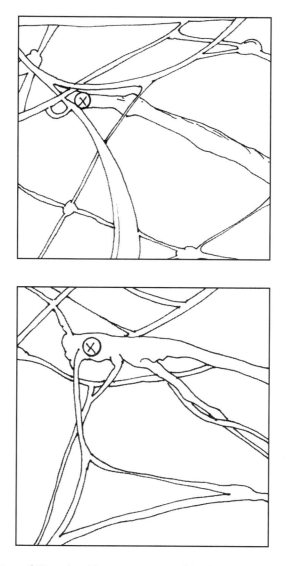

Fig. 42 and Fig. 43 Changing microfibrils, 3 seconds apart

EXPLORATION 47: TUNING TO YOUR MICROFIBRIL DANCE

Find a comfortable place to lie down and settle into your body. Let your body relax and feel the sensation of temperature, texture and pressure on your skin.

Bring your awareness through the outside surface of skin and feel the blood-side of skin. Notice the warm, fluid, spongy nature of the area and move through it with your mind's eye until you find the superficial layers of the fascial matrix. Notice their distinct layer of fibers and fluid. Imagine your microfibrils connected to a lattice, as well as stretching between nerves, blood vessels and tissue into deeper layers.

Now imagine you are a microscope and see into this layer, distinguishing between the fibers, fluid and cells in the matrix. Bring your awareness to the collagen fibers. Let your microscope see into the microfibrils. Move your awareness to the spaces between the microfibrils and notice the rippling, vibrating organized water inside.

From the water-filled spaces between the microfibrils, begin to feel the movement of your wave pattern as it vibrates throughout these spaces. Imagine you can travel through them. Shift your body position while keeping your awareness inside the water-filled spaces. Notice the dance between your microfibrils.

Move back out from the organized water into the microfibrils, into the collagen fibers, into the fascia, to the blood-side of skin, and out to the outside of skin. Notice the sensations at the skin. Feel the difference in your proprioception and the feeling of depth in the body.

LIQUID CRYSTALLINE MATRIX: MUTABILITY AND STABILITY

The liquid ground substance and intercellular fluid create a stable medium for the microfibril movement. This combination of stability and mutability creates consistency and integration while giving the body an amazing capacity to adapt to the internal and external environments. Because of this combination our bodies are able to be a closed system where energy is continually recirculating within the liquid crystalline matrix. It is an ideal way for our bodies to function in a changing environment without diminishing our potency and quality of energy.

THE LIQUID CRYSTALLINE MATRIX AND AGING

When the crystalline matrix is both stable and mutable, it's able to respond to the environment efficiently and effectively. As we develop and move through our life, the activities we engage in, along with our relationship to gravity, creates habitual repetitive movement patterns and constant pressure in our bodies. These patterns create tensile and contractive repetitive responses that, along with crosslinking and chemical changes, limit the ability of our microfibrils to shift and change. This patterning helps the body move along habitual lines. We use this crystal memory, as well as neurological patterning, to move us without our mind needing to participate.

As we age this repetitive memory patterning slowly reduces the complexity and mutability of the microfibril/organized water matrix. This in turn reduces our range and diversity of movement and creates inertial patterns. It over-stabilizes the system, so when you begin to move, the fascial matrix resists the movement instead of shifting with the movement. The older you are, the more this becomes apparent… especially when you first get up and try to move. As you warm the tissue with movement and activate the ionic forces of the fascial matrix, the microfibrils begin to respond to the inputs. Because of the rigidity in the matrix, it is hard for the body to relate to gravity through the midline. Instead we count on the strain and shearing forces on the body to hold us. This limits our sense of balance and deteriorates the tissue's resilience, potent vitality.

This stiffness, lack of balance and difficulty in initiating movement can be reversed by taking time to move the microfibril/organized water matrix in new and different ways. If we are aware of our body's limitations and begin to move in different, nonfunctional ways, then we can begin to open up the fascial system to recalibrate its bioelectric matrix. Put another way, we can begin to move from the conductive wave motion in our organized water instead of from our patterned matrix. As we reintroduce spiraling, vibrating and pulsating movements into our fascial matrix, starting at the neutral place of the midline, we enliven our conductive interconnected bodies. (See Chapter 22: Self-practice).

LIQUID CRYSTALLINE MATRIX AND TOUCH

We can connect our own crystalline matrix to another person's matrix through touch, which is one of the reasons touch is so important in our lives. When we touch another person, our crystalline fascial matrix reaches out to touch and entangle with their matrix. As the healthy aspects of our respective matrices begin to move together, information is exchanged between them, entraining wave patterns and connecting our balanced reciprocal tensions. One person may impulse into the other's matrix system, activating the microfibrils to rearrange and reintegrate in beneficial ways.

When we consciously activate the microfibril/organized water matrix through touch, we unwind its memory patterns, reconnect and complexify its relationships, and bring greater adaptability to the system. This in turn activates microfibrils, and the full circle of exchange continues. Bodyworkers like to say that when you give a massage, you should feel like you *received* a massage as well. This comes from the exchange between the two liquid crystalline matrices.

This explains one of the underlying benefits and functions of massage, bodywork, acupuncture, homeopathy, chiropractic work and other impulse-driven therapies for both client and practitioner. While we are using the neurological system to understand, decide, distinguish and determine, we are also using our liquid crystalline matrix to connect, communicate and exchange.

EXPLORATION 48: TOUCHING AND DANCING WITH THE LIQUID CRYSTALLINE MATRIX (WITH A PARTNER)

Have your partner lie on their back on a massage table or bed and settle into their body. Sit to the side of them and settle into your own body.

Bring your awareness to your hands and find the microfibril/organized water matrix in your palms. Feel the connection to your whole matrix and notice how it is rippling, vibrating and conducting throughout your body. Bring your awareness back to your hands and feel your microfibrils coming to the surface of your palm, connecting to the currents in the external environment. Feel how the attention of your fascial matrix moves toward the surface of your hands.

Now place one hand palm up under your partner's torso, and one hand palm down on top of the torso, keeping both hands in line with one other. Settle your hands into the body. Let your hands connect to the microfibril/organized water matrix of your partner.

Notice or imagine the pull of coherence as your microfibrils connect. Feel the small, subtle, rippling, vibrating waters in your partner's liquid crystalline matrix.

Feel how your two wave patterns become a single, rippling conduction pattern. When you feel the crystalline matrix of your partner move, follow that movement with your whole matrix. Let your whole body dance with that movement. Keep your hands connected to your partner's matrix. Don't move your palms across the skin of your partner, but move with the internal matrix. Feel the fluidity and wave patterns in the liquid coherence.

As you dance with your partner's liquid crystalline matrix, let the healing, coherent crystalline nature of the matrix inform and heal your cells and tissue.

When you feel a pause of a deep stillness in your partner's matrix, gently lift your hands and disengage from your partner's matrix. Now let your internal matrix glide and move, reintegrating your own crystalline matrix. Feel the shift in your own body and ask your partner to share their experience.

CHAPTER 11

THE BODY'S FRACTAL DESIGN

The human body is designed to respond or connect in multiple directions. The directions written in your body's DNA allow our tissues to develop, grow and maintain themselves by dividing body structures from larger to smaller in a self-similar pattern. In our fascia, the hollow conducting tubes of our microfibrils are patterned after the microtubules inside our cells and continue outward to the larger pattern in our collagen fibers. These similar patterns—from microscopic cytoskeletons to microfibril to collagen fibers—resonate and relate within us, integrating our micro- and macro-levels of structure. This type of design is fractal in nature, in that its structure divides mathematically to smaller and smaller sizes, maintaining the same shape and capacity. Fractal design is seen throughout nature and in all living things.

WHAT IS A FRACTAL DESIGN?

A *fractal design* is formed through a mathematical formula of algorithms that creates an amazingly self-similar pattern from the largest to the smallest part. This pattern repeats itself on scales of size, forming similar structures at every level. There are many examples of fractal design in nature, including the branching of a trees, blood vessels and snowflakes.

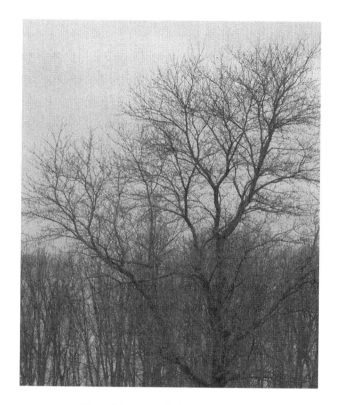

Fig. 44 Fractal design in tree

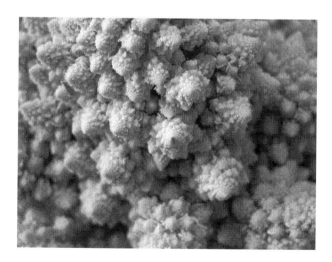

Fig. 45 Fractal design in Cauliflower

The fractal design in our fascia comes from the arrangement of collagen fibers in the matrix continuing as a self-similar pattern to the arrangements within and among the microfibrils. This pattern of branching in the collagen fibers and microfibrils is maintained as the individual fibers connect and reconnect when we move and shift our relationship to gravity. Even with this constant shifting, the fractal design maintains integrity, holding to the fractal relationship in nature.

Charles Ridley: "Fractals describe the ever-repeating "self-similar" patterns of life that are nested within one another, and fractal theory recognizes the relationship between the whole patterns and the patterns of all its parts. Nature utilizes living fractal geometry to create living organisms."

–From *Stillness: Biodynamic Cranial Practice and the Evolution of Consciousness*, **North Atlantic Books, pg. 193.**

FRACTAL COLLAGEN FIBERS TO MICROFIBRILS

We can see how our microfibrils are nested in our collagen fibers by looking at different levels of magnification. Collagen fibers have a resonant relationship, shifting and changing in self similar patterns from the smallest part the largest part, and maintaining their fractal design. Because such a fractal design is seen in all connective tissues, as well as in all cells, this geometry is interconnected throughout the body. The ability of our different tubular structures to structure and organize water, create a bioelectric matrix, and shift in self similar patterns gives our bodies an inclusive fractal matrix whereby all of our cells are able to communicate.

This integrated, conductive framework is where many scientists now theorize our consciousness and awareness reside.

EXPLORATION 49: FINDING OUR FRACTAL DESIGN

Find a comfortable sitting position and settle into your body. Let your awareness focus on your whole body and its tubular nature of arms, legs, long muscles and spine.

Bring awareness to your fascial matrix and notice its tubular nature, surrounding arms and legs, long muscles, viscera and spinal cord. Let your awareness move into your fascial matrix and notice your collagen fibers. Feel the tubular nature of these fibers and their connections with each other.

Go to the microscopic level of your collagen fibers and notice the microfibrils within your collagen fibers. Notice the fluid within and between these tubular structures.

Bring your awareness to your cells and notice the tubular nature of the cytoskeleton. Notice this connected matrix inside the cell and how it branches and connects out to the cells around it.

Now find your way back from the cells' cytoskeleton, microfibrils, collagen fibers and whole body.

Come back to stillness and notice the different sensations you experience in your body.

FRACTAL COMPLEXITY

The fractal design of the various tubular structures in our bodies is complex and dynamic. The arrangement and rearrangement of the fractal matrix creates an interconnected web that is designed to adapt to the pressures and tensions of our internal and external environments. This three-dimensional complexity allows our body to navigate in the world smoothly and easily without friction or resistance.

This fractal complexity also allows our body to maintain function and form. The pace and stress of our lives is continually testing this matrix, pushing and pulling, shifting fractal relationships, and creating inertial patterns in the body.

We can directly affect this fractal arrangement by contacting the fractal matrix. When we put a linear impulse into the matrix, whether through movement or hands-on techniques, we create a shift in the fractal arrangement. Because of the fractal complexity, the impulse will move immediately throughout the whole matrix too fast for us to follow. In order for us to maintain this fractal design in the matrix, shifts and changes throughout the system are geared to balance around the midline, maintaining equilibrium.

Charles Ridley: "Any intervention… produces body-wide effects in the client. Therefore, each linear change I make to the client's body initiates a body-wide fractal adaptation that either decreases or increases stress in his or her bodymind."

–From *Stillness: Biodynamic Cranial Practice and the Evolution of Consciousness*, North Atlantic Books, pg. 5.

LINEAR VS. MULTIDIRECTIONAL IMPULSE

When we work with the fractal design of the fascia we understand that each impulse brings a whole-body response through our fractal matrix. When we use a linear impulse, whether through a vector of movement or through touch, we limit our influence within the direction of that vector. This impulse is felt by our whole body matrix, and it responds to that directional vector. When we use a multidirectional impulse through varied movement or multiple points of contact, we give our matrix a three-dimensional space in which to respond. This initiates an unwinding of the area as well as a whole-body response.

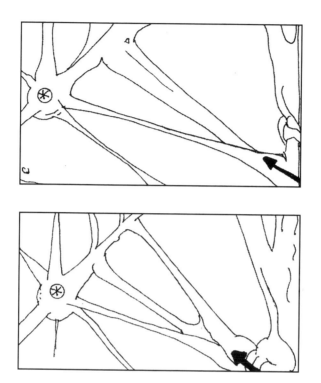

Fig. 46a and Fig. 46b Linear pulse

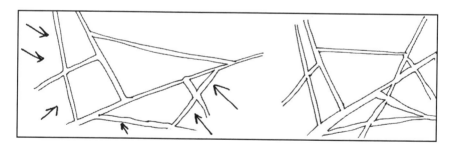

Fig. 47 Multidirectional pulse

EXPLORATION 50: LINEAR AND MULTIDIRECTIONAL IMPULSES

Find a comfortable place to lie down and settle into your body. Bring your awareness to your fascial matrix and focus on its fractal design of tubular structures as it gets smaller and smaller. Feel the tubule matrix as a moving, rippling, interconnected design in a sea of fluid. Imagine this tubule matrix like entangled seaweed floating in the ocean currents.

Begin by gently and slowly flexing and extending one foot, feeling the longitudinal glide in the fractal matrix in your leg. Let your awareness to the different levels of the matrix in your fascia and in your cells, feeling how all levels are moving. Repeat with other foot.

Now create a horizontal impulse into the fractal matrix in your leg by gently pulling toward the inside of the leg and then to the outside of the leg. Let your awareness move from the whole matrix to the microfibrils, feeling how all of the levels in the matrix are moving. Repeat with other leg.

Now create a multidirectional impulse by placing your heel on the floor and gently and slowly make a figure eight with the foot, starting at the toes, moving up and around and down the arch to the heel, then moving down and around. Feel how the whole matrix of the leg is gliding in a multidirectional way. Let your awareness move from the whole matrix of the microfibrils, feeling how all levels of the matrix are moving in this pattern. Repeat with other foot.

Come back to stillness and notice the different sensation in your feet and legs. Let your matrix move, integrating the shifts in your lower extremities.

FRACTALS AND THE LEMNISCATE

One patterned rhythm that is found in the fractal landscape of the body is the *lemniscate*. The lemniscate is basically the pattern of a figure eight or the infinity symbol. In the living organism it is a flow of relationship that can move in many directions and shapes, always flowing back into itself by looping back and forth. The center point of this figure eight is the point of stillness between the cycles of moving in and out. The midline of the body is this still point for the wave pulsations that move in a figure eight around the spine. The three-dimensional lemniscate design is the pattern that allows external input to move into the body and internal input to move to the outer body. This pattern is the how information is exchanged in the body and out of the body.

EXPLORATION 51: MOVING THE LEMNISCATE AROUND YOUR MIDLINE

Sit in a chair facing the back of the chair and your feet on the floor on either side of the seat. Let your arms rest on the back of the chair. Find the midline in the center of your torso and let your body relax into your center line.

Gently begin a small movement out from the midline to the side of your body and then back to the midline. Keep your spine straight and don't bend from side to side. This is a small spreading out from the center line and back.

Now starting at the neck, gently move out from the center of your spine to one side and then turn that movement back into the center of your spine in a loop. Take that loop to the other side with a gentle glide out, around and back. This is a figure eight lemniscate.

Continue down your back with slow, gliding movements in this figure eight pattern. Let the figure eight just move around the spine. Let the figure eight move out to the side of the body.

Change the direction of the figure eight so that it loops around to the front of the torso and then to the back. Create a flower of figure eight loops around a center point at the spine.

Come back to stillness and feel the information flow around the spine.

FRACTALS AND COHERENCE

The fractal design throughout our fascia gives our tissue the ability to resonate through the self-similar patterns from macro- to micro-levels. This creates a dynamic, coherent equilibrium that maintains the organization of our organism. This coherent, organized energy relationship creates vitality, potency and adaptability for our body. Our level of health determines, and is determined by, our coherent equilibrium. When our whole-body coherence is impaired, our fractal arrangements collapse and our communication networks are disconnected.

Charles Ridley: "The subsequent breakdown in health transfers chaos to the bodymind matrix that breaks up the fractal organization, and the coherent equilibrium collapses."

–From *Stillness: Biodynamic Cranial Practice and the Evolution of Consciousness*, North Atlantic Books, pg. 5.

FRACTALS AND CHAOS THEORY

In the realm of quantum physics, nature is viewed as a chaotic system. Different from classical physics, where order and predictability reigns, *chaos theory* understands the ability of the natural living world to adapt and change to input from its surroundings. In chaos theory, systems have a determining equation ruling behavior, are sensitive to their initial development, and beneath their random behavior there is a sense of order. Chaos theory reflects how we as a living organism are able to be a whole system and simultaneously allow for autonomy within the different functioning layers of our bodies. This is created through the fractal design within the body.

Mae-Wan Ho, Ph.D: "This has led to the discovery that healthy rhythms exhibit deterministic chaos and fractal self-similarity, reflecting the constant communication between different biological rhythms that takes place in a healthy, coherent organism."

–From *The Rainbow and the Worm: The Physics of Organisms*, World Scientific, pg. 287.

EXPLORATION 52: FRACTAL DESIGN AND COHERENCE

Find a comfortable place to lie down and settle into your body. Bring your awareness to your fascial matrix. Let your focus move from your whole matrix to your collagen fibers, then to your microfibrils, to the cytoskeleton of your cells, and finally to your fractal design.

Let your matrix begin to gently move and glide. Feel the interconnectedness in all the levels of your matrix. Notice how they all respond to the glide at the same time but in their own way. Feel the gliding, waving motion of the tubules within the surrounding fluid, like waves of seaweed in the ocean.

Now bring your awareness to the functions of your body. Notice your breath bringing air in and out. Notice your heart pumping the blood. Notice your digestive system moving nourishment into your system and removing toxins from your system.

Now overlay the functioning and the wave motion of the fractal layers. Feel the coherence underneath all these different biological rhythms.

Shift your focus back to gliding your internal matrix, continuing to feel the underlying coherence. Come to stillness and notice the different sensations in your body.

CHAPTER 12
BIOTENSEGRITY

WHAT IS TENSEGRITY?

Tensegrity, derived from the words tension and integrity, is a structure that is composed of isolated, compressed parts inside a webbing of continuous tension. The compressed parts—usually bars, triangles, crosses or icosahedrons—are suspended in a webbing of cables that are pulled taut to create space and stability for the compressed parts. These cables stretch out to meet the external pressure of gravity and the atmosphere, equalizing and transferring the external pressure along the surface of the structure.

The structure is self-stabilizing, transferring any external forces throughout the structure, creating flexibility and integrity. Because the structure is "pre-stressed" it can resume its original shape after being pushed and pulled by external forces. The structure is also lightweight but strong, because of its continuous tension (suspension) and discontinuous compression (coherence).

Does this sound familiar? Tensegrity is seen in many structures, macro and micro, in our living world. Our fascial structure, with its suspension and coherence, is one example of a living tensegrity structure.

These aspects of tensegrity apply to the structural architecture of the body and nature. Dr. Stephen M Levin, an orthopedic surgeon and former Associate Professor at Michigan State University created the term *Biotensegrity* 40 years ago, referring to the tensegrity structure of tensile and compressive forces within the body. He has written papers including *The icosahedron as a biolog-*

ical support system, Primordial Structure and Conscious Tension, Discontinuous Compression: A Model for Biomechanical Support of the Body. He organized the first Biotensegrity Summit in September, 2015 in Washington D.C.

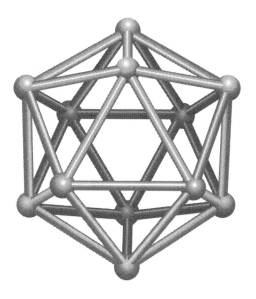

Fig. 48 Tensegrity Model

Sondra Barrett, Ph.D.: "Tensegrity: Refers to any physical structure that stabilizes and supports itself by balancing forces of tension and contraction. Structures are stabilized mechanically by balancing internal and external forces."

–From *Secrets of Your Cells: Discovering Your Body's Inner Intelligence*, Sounds True, pg.74.

TENSEGRITY TO BIOTENSEGRITY

The term tensegrity comes from the work of architect-futurist Buckminster Fuller. Fuller used this tensile integrity to create physical structures, including his famous geodesic domes. These structures were lightweight yet extremely strong, due to the balancing tension and compressions created by the struts, cables and triangular designs in the dome. They are known to be one of the most stable architectural designs.

Buckminster Fuller was a great observer of nature's own structure, looking at the smallest parts like atoms and cells, to larger phenomena like trees, solar systems and galaxies. He saw how the solid parts in many structures were all held in place by a continuous and flexible webbing, allowing them to be independent and stable while adapting to the external forces of the environment. Our fascia (the webbing) and our organs (solid parts) mimic this structure, as do many other relationships in our body.

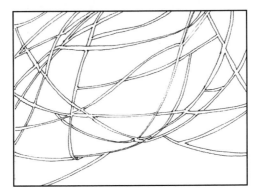

Fig. 49 Continuous flexible webbing

Dr. Donald Ingber, a Senior Associate in Pathology and Surgery of Vascular Biology at Harvard Medical School, whose exposure to Fuller's structural design in an art class, led him to realize that the cell had tensegrity structural components within its cytoskeleton. He discovered how the body uses tensegrity to build the cell and interconnect it with the nucleus and out into the extracellular matrix. He recognized how this structure creates a strong and flexible body, as well as a responsive interconnected body. Dr. Ingber also showed how this structure was able to transmit the external forces on the surface of the cell into the nucleus, which created biochemical changes, activating or deactivating genes.

Dr. Ingber referred to this as *mechanotransduction*, and he went on to show how this response to pressure and force influenced the growth, configuration and function of the cells, tissues and organs.

Sondra Barrett, PhD: "At a biological level, tensegrity allows us to comprehend how changes in shape and mechanical strain influence cellular choices and actions."

–From *Secrets of Your Cells: Discovering Your Body's Inner Intelligence*, Sounds True, pg. 75.

This bridge from architectural structures to nature's structures created a breakthrough in our understanding and use of the term tensegrity. We now understand that tensegrity's powerful capacity to create structures that are adaptive to their environment, self-stabilizing and independent (yet interconnected) is a natural prerequisite for any living organism.

This brought new explanations for how the body deals with the external forces of gravity and pressure. We now understand that instead of a structure defined by axial-loaded compression—i.e., built on the blocks of vertebra and the strength of the bones—we are in fact a structure defined by continuous tension and discontinuous compression, where the bones are suspended in soft tissue. This allows us to be independent yet interactive with gravity.

Taking these ideas a step further, Dr. Steve Levin, an orthopedic surgeon, created the term *biotensegrity* to describe the tensegrity concept in biological organisms. He applied it to the human body where the tensile forces, are the fascia and muscles, and the discontinuous compression forces are the bones. This balanced reciprocal tension creates the ability of the body to glide and suspend through the gravitational forces we live in.

The fascial matrix is a microscopic fractal of the body's biotensegrity. This biotensegrity gives us the capacity to glide through space, defy gravity, have individual and interconnected functions go on at the same time, and tap into the information network that allows our body to work as one organism.

Dr. Stephen Levin: "Tensegrity icosahedrons are used to model biologic organisms from viruses to vertebrates, their cells, systems and subsystems. There are only tension and compression elements in tensegrity systems. There are no shears, bending moments or levers, just simple tension and compression, in a self-organizing, hierarchical, load distributing, low energy consuming structure."

–From Steve Levin's website: http//www.biotensegrity.com/

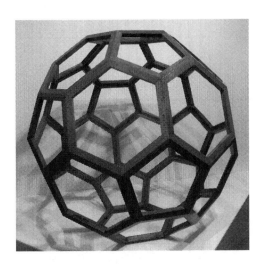

Fig. 50 Truncated Icosahedron

When looking under the microscope, Jean-Claude Guimberteau, MD, a hand surgeon and medical researcher, discovered the amazing microfibril matrix within the superficial fascia under the skin. As he spread out the living tissue, you can see, in a series of videos, the icosahedron vacuoles that hold the tensegrity structure of the hand together. You can also see how vacuoles shift and change when pressure is applied to them. When you release the pressure, the icosahedrons reconfigure to fill the space with the matrix. The videos "Strolling Under the Skin" and "The architecture of life" that Dr. Guimberteau produced have changed the way we understand the biotensegrity matrix.

EXPLORATION 53: FINDING YOUR BIOTENSEGRITY

Find a comfortable place to lie down and settle into your body. Bring your awareness to your fascial matrix.

Focus on your superficial fascia lying just below the skin. Feel its wholeness. Feel its compressive nature as it holds all of your tissues and organs inside. Feel its tensile nature as it stretches around bones, organs and tissues.

Spread your fingers apart, feeling the tensile factors expanding but holding the matrix intact. Then let your fingers relax, feeling the compressive factors holding the matrix, returning the fingers to a neutral position.

Inhale and exhale slowly and deeply. Feel how your internal matrix spreads and expands, then glides back. Feel the tensile and compressive forces shift with your internal movement while also continuing to hold the space for your lungs and heart.

Now let you matrix glide and move, staying focused on the tensile and compressive forces as they are engaged in the glide.

Come back to stillness and feel the support and buoyancy of your internal matrix.

QUALITIES OF TENSEGRITY STRUCTURES IN THE BODY

- Continuous tension, discontinuous compression
- Self-stabilizing
- Pre-stressed
- Resilient
- Pressure at one point felt by whole structure
- Interconnection between tensegrity structures
- Fractal in the body

TENSEGRITY IN CELLS

Tensegrity is found in the intercellular matrix of the cytoskeleton. This tensile structure creates the shape, stability and space so the structures inside the cell can function independently. The cytoskeleton of the cell is made of actomyosin microtubules that connect the nucleus to the cell membrane and to the extracellular tensegrity structure, essentially interconnecting all the cells of the body.

Sondra Barrett, Ph.D.: "This cytoskeleton matrix transports molecules, coordinates information and regulates genetic expression. With the ability to balance the push-pull of the cell, it is the newest biological candidate for the seat of cellular intelligence as well as the seat of consciousness."

–**From** *Secrets of Your Cells: Discovering Your Body's Inner Intelligence*, **Sounds True, pg. 77.**

From the molecular level, this tensegrity structure can be seen in the attractive and repulsive forces of the ions in the protein-based cytoskeleton. At the quantum level, this tensegrity creates the structure for the quantum coherence that is found in living organisms.

TENSEGRITY IN THE FASCIA

Tensegrity in the fascia is fractal in nature, from the tensile and compressive forces (1) between the fascia and the solid structures in the body, (2) between the collagen fibers and solid structures in the fascial webbing and (3) between the microfibrils and organized water. The balanced tension between ionic forces creates this tensile and compressive relationship on the molecular level. This tensegrity throughout the fascial system gives space, stability and shape to our body, while shifting around the balanced reciprocal tension in the structure. This tensegrity structure is interconnected with other tensegrity relationships between our bones, ligaments, tendons, muscles and cells.

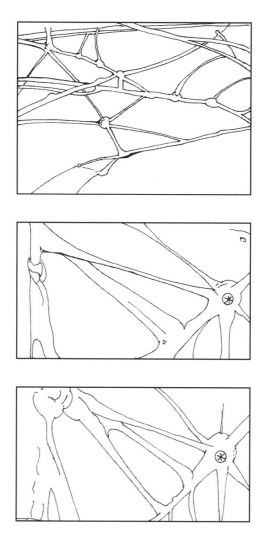

Fig. 51, Fig 52a, and Fig. 52b Biotensegrity structure in Fascia

FLOATING COMPRESSION

Floating compression is another description of tensegrity coined by Kenneth Snelson. He is an artist who uses tensegrity to create sculptures that demonstrate suspension in space. His sculptures demonstrate the ability of tensegrity structures to suspend compressed parts so that outside forces do not impede their ability to function. His work gives us a better understanding of how the

167

bones, organs and cells can suspend in the fascial matrix while functioning efficiently, not being pulled down by gravity.

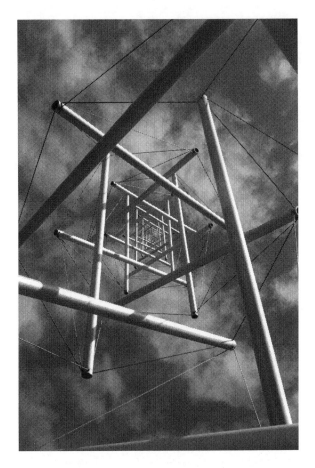

Fig. 53 Floating Compression

CHAPTER 13

FIBER CONNECTIONS

CELL MATRIX FIBERS

Inside our cell membrane there are three kinds of fiber structures that make up the cytoskeleton of each cell. They consist of microtubules (the largest, that are made of the protein tubulin), actin microfilaments (the smallest, that are made of the protein actin), and midsize microfilaments (made of a combination of proteins). Although they have different functions in our cells, these three fiber structures all provide structure and support to the cell, help in cell division, provide transport for certain elements in the cell, and connect the internal cellular environment to the external environment.

In this book we are most interested in the connection between the microtubules in our cells and the microfibrils in our fascia. Although the microtubules are made of different proteins than those of microfibrils, they have the same capacity to conduct through the organized water within and surrounding them. This conductive capacity gives our body—from cells, to fascia, to the outside world—the ability to communicate vibration and wave patterns coherently throughout our fiber networks.

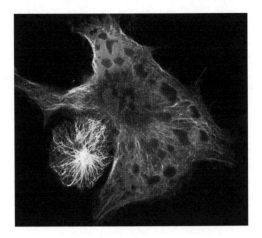

Fig. 54 Microtubules in Cell

FASCIAL MATRIX FIBERS

Within our fascial ground substance, fascial fibers vary in relationship to function. They are all created by the fibroblasts, using collagen protein to form the protocollagen fibers, microfibrils and collagen fibers. Although there are many different kinds of collagen, they all have a repeating sequence of the amino acids glycine and proline, which line up head to tail and side by side, creating long fibrils that thicken into microfibrils and collagen fibers.

Some of our collagen fibers merge into tendon or muscle tissues, adding actin filaments to respond to the contractive forces of movement. These filaments can also be seen attaching to joint capsules, ligaments and other soft tissues, where strong push and pull forces need stronger attachments.

Our fascia also creates retinacular cutis fibers that connect layers of fascia. These can vary in thickness and flexibility, restricting movement. This can be a positive functional adaptation, for example in our hands and feet. Or it can be in the form of adhesions that respond to forces of imbalance, inertial patterns, or excess pull and compression.

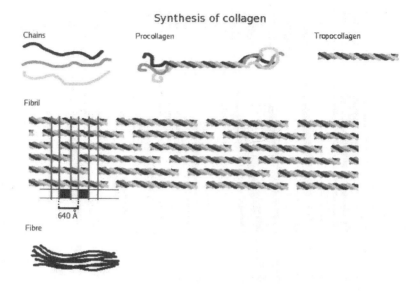

Fig. 55 Collagen Fibers in Fascia

Throughout this book, I have used the terms fascial matrix, bioelectric matrix and liquid crystalline matrix interchangeably to describe this microfibril/organized water matrix of fascia that conducts wave patterns through its watery spaces. As we have seen, this bioelectric crystalline matrix allows for immediate, rapid communication through our whole body. Some scientists are now theorizing that the liquid crystalline matrix is the seat of consciousness and awareness in the body. This ability to create a cooperative interrelationship and order within us gives the microtubule/microfibril/organized water matrix the ability to be consciously aware of our wholeness without a central controlling agent.

EXPLORATION 54: CONNECTING OUR LIQUID CRYSTALLINE MATRIX FROM CELL TO FASCIA TO WORLD

Find a comfortable place to lie down and settle into your body. Bring your awareness to your internal matrix. Focus on your superficial layer, feeling the coherence in your whole body. Move through your middle layers, feeling the spaces between your organs and other tissues. Focus on the deepest level of your matrix inside your vertebrae around your spinal cord. Feel the coherence around the spine and up into the membranes in the head.

Stay connected to all the layers of your matrix and shift to the micro-level of your microfibrils and the organized water surrounding them. Feel the coherence and conductivity in the water within your microfibrils. Focus on this liquid crystalline matrix, feeling the rippling, vibrating wave motion within your matrix.

Shift your awareness to your cells. Notice the cytoskeleton within the membrane of your cells. Feel the microtubule matrix in your cytoskeleton and feel its coherence within the cells. Feel how the matrix inside your cells reaches out from its coherence and touches the microfibril/organized water matrix in your fascia.

Follow the connections from your microtubules to your microfibrils, and then to your different layers of fascia.

Feel the microfibrils below the skin reaching out to the electromagnetic field of the external environment. Feel your coherent connection to the larger organism of Earth.

Disengage from the external field and settle into your own matrix. Notice how the sensation of your coherent wholeness has changed.

CHAPTER 14
COHERENT AWARENESS, CONSCIOUSNESS AND THE MATRIX

Mae-Wan Ho, Ph.D: "Body consciousness possessing all the hallmarks of consciousness–sentience, intercommunication and memory–is distributed throughout the entire liquid crystalline matrix that connects each cell to every other. Brain consciousness associated with the nervous system is embedded in body consciousness and is coupled to it."

–From *The Rainbow and the Worm: The Physics of Organisms*, World Scientific, pg. 237.

BRAIN CONSCIOUSNESS, BODY CONSCIOUSNESS, MATRIX CONSCIOUSNESS

Consciousness is the state of being awake and aware of one's self and one's surroundings. Most of science has looked to the nervous system and the synapsing of a complex matrix of nerve cells as the place where consciousness provides us with sensations, feelings and perceptions that we use to understand and act in our lives. This brain consciousness fuels our thoughts, desires and actions in the world. When we are awake and aware of inputs from our external and internal environment, our nervous system interacts with the information, filters it through our complex memory and safety systems and reacts accordingly. This mind processing connects us with the external world and is the engine that drives our experience.

Brain consciousness uses awareness to distinguish between the self and everything else. It gives us the foundation from which our determination of safety and survival depend on. It gives us the perception of separateness and holds the boundary between ourselves and others.

Then how are we able to be fully aware of ourselves as a living organism not separate from the "big" organism? How do we maintain the awareness of our relationship to the whole as the mind propels us forward through time? And how does this kind of awareness change our propensity to be guided by the survival mechanisms of our autonomic nervous system? This ability to maintain awareness, experience the integrated living system of the big organism and not react to the survival and safety cues of our autonomic nervous system comes from the consciousness of the internal matrix. The consciousness of the internal matrix (the liquid crystalline matrix), can be divided into body consciousness and matrix consciousness.

Body consciousness is the ability to embody our personal experience. It is the state of awareness that senses and feels our integrated moving, changing system. It is the state of being awake and aware of ourselves in relationship to our physical environment. You may have experienced embodiment when you feel safe, settled, grounded and connected to yourself and your environment. You may have noticed embodiment in others who are centered, grounded and at home in their bodies. Body consciousness is an integral and dominant part of most wild animals that inhabit the earth. As modern, mind centered animals, we have let brain consciousness dominate our experience.

Matrix consciousness is the state of being aware of the whole integrated system undifferentiated from the environment. It holds the "felt sense" of being alive, with no drive to become or act. It provides a sense of coherence, presence and interconnectedness both internally and externally. It provides the cues to experience the fractal connections from cells, to organism, to environment, to biosphere as undifferentiated. It is the state of no judgement, no desire and no separation. It is the place we experience in meditation, in being present, in deep connection. The elements of safety and survival are not relevant to the consciousness of the matrix.

Body consciousness and brain consciousness can interface to provide us with the tools to experience our aliveness and interconnectedness as well as respond to the complexity of our world. When we cultivate matrix consciousness we can rest in the wholeness of the big organism, letting the relationship between ourselves and the rest of the world shift and change through the balanced reciprocal tensions of life.

COHERENT MATRIX

Although scientists have linked consciousness to the brain and our thinking mind, this belief disregards the "felt sense" experience, the mindfulness experience of the present moment and the undifferentiated self. When we meditate and suspend thinking, we enter into a different space of awareness and consciousness.

Scientists have begun to discover that other parts of the living organism besides the nervous system have the capacity of awareness and consciousness. With the help of quantum physics, the concept of coherence has been used to describe what makes something alive and conscious. This quantum coherence is found inside the tubular fibers where organized water (liquid crystalline matrix) creates a conductive pathway throughout our body. This liquid crystalline matrix may be the source of our ability to take the separate pieces of the body and mind, and unite them into a conscious being. The coherence of the matrix, from the microtubules of the cell to the microfibrils of the connective tissue, to the electromagnetic field around the earth gives us the felt sense of wholeness, integration and interconnectedness. This coherence in the matrix is where matrix consciousness resides just like brain consciousness resides in the nervous system.

This matrix consciousness through its coherent matrix takes us down a completely different experiential road than brain consciousness of the nervous system. It also creates abilities beyond the scope of the nervous system.

MATRIX CONSCIOUSNESS AND ACTIVITY

The integration of consciousness, memory, sensory input and patterning allows us to perform many activities without needing to relearn them each time.

Many of our activities are complex and need immediate response from our sensory motor systems. For example, the hand-eye coordination, memory and fine motor skills needed to play a difficult piano concerto require an amazing coherence of all our systems. The nervous system is not equipped to send signals quickly enough to and from the brain and hands to play complex piano pieces. This coherent ability must come from some other source.

Dr. Guimbierto , the French hand surgeon who used a microscope to observe the microfibrils of the fascial matrix, shows in his videos how the microfibrils under the skin shift and change to allow fast, smooth coordinated movement in the hands playing the piano. He asks the question as to how the hands can move in this complex way and then return to their original state when they are still. He points to the microfibril/organized water matrix as the answer.

This coherent ability of the body to effortlessness move in complex ways integrates the nervous system of consciousness and the coherent awareness in the microfibril/organized water matrix of consciousness. This coherent awareness is a felt sense in the matrix that gives us a different conscious experience of ourselves and our surroundings. This conscious awareness does not follow the nerve pathways that create safety, demand understanding and propel our responses. It emerges as an integrated, whole body (matrix) felt sense of wellbeing and interconnectedness.

Consciousness through the nervous system propels us into relationship with ourselves and the world. Coherent awareness through the microfibril/organized water allows us to experience the coherent wholeness of our being. The two together determine our adaptability, vitality, health and wellbeing.

CONSCIOUSNESS AND SURVIVAL

Because our brain consciousness propels action, it has become the dominant player in how we experience our lives. Brain consciousness interfaces with the somatic and autonomic nervous systems. The autonomic nervous system is regulated by our sense of safety and survival, using memory cues to create fear responses in the central nervous system. This fear/survival perception creates a cascade of reactions through the nervous system and diminishes the influence of our body and matrix consciousness. Because we experience many traumas (both large and small) in a lifetime, this fear/survival response memory can dominate our daily experience and response to life. As this overrides our body and matrix consciousness, we begin to have pathological, psychological unconscious responses to perceived threats.

Without the input of body and matrix consciousness, our world becomes more separate and isolated by the need to respond to threat. We stay protected and isolated perceiving everything outside of ourselves as potential safety threats.

When we cultivate body and matrix consciousness we begin to reinstate the awareness and experience of interconnectedness. We shift our experience from the polarity of differences to the relationship of similarities. We shift from perceiving life as a series of threatening encounters to a synergistic flow of interrelated experiences. This shifts us from the "us and them" consciousness to the "we" consciousness.

So, how do we make this shift in consciousness? We use our conscious brain and body awareness to shift our attention to the coherent awareness of matrix consciousness.

CONSCIOUS AWARENESS AND COHERENT AWARENESS

Conscious awareness is the state of being aware of our sensations and feelings through our body's nervous system. As we spend time in conscious awareness we can differentiate sensations, know the different qualities of feelings and begin to understand what propels our perceptions and thoughts. The more we spend time in conscious awareness, the more we experience the complexity of our lives. If we let go of this conscious awareness and let it propel us into action, we can see the consequences (positive and negative) of our complex awareness. Conscious awareness perceives the different pieces of information that inform our choices. Conscious awareness tunes to the different parts of us that create a unified, individual system.

Coherent awareness is the state of being aware of the relationship between our wholeness and the wholeness of the planet. As we spend time in coherent awareness, we develop the felt sense of our interconnectedness to all living things. The more we spend time in coherent awareness, the more we experience the undifferentiated self and the ebb and flow of the universe. Coherent awareness perceives the interrelationship of everything, Coherent awareness tunes us to the interconnectedness between the individual self and the universe.

FORMLESS AWARENESS

When we cultivate coherent awareness, we have to suspend the louder voices of brain consciousness. We first have to quiet the mind from its endless responses to brain consciousness and settle into body consciousness. As we allow ourselves to quiet the brain's activities we begin to shift our awareness to the coherent awareness of the internal matrix. Meditation, mindfulness, relaxation, listening to music and being in nature foster our cultivation of coherent awareness. Activities which takes us past the thinking process, such as running in the "zone" or playing a complex music piece, cultivate coherent awareness.

In the Buddhist tradition, cultivating mindfulness and formal meditation take us into the experience of *formless awareness.* This formless awareness is the coherent

EXPLORATION 55: EXPERIENCING COHERENT AWARENESS THROUGH YOUR MATRIX

Find a comfortable place to lie down and settle into your body. Bring your awareness to your internal matrix. Shift your focus into the microscopic view of your microfibrils in the fascial matrix and your microtubules in the cellular matrix. Notice how they are interconnected. Visualize the organized water pathways between the fibers. Use your felt sense to experience this interconnected matrix as whole and undifferentiated. Notice the experience of body consciousness.

Now bring your awareness to your breath. Breathe in and out normally. When your mind shifts its focus to a thought or other activity, gently bring it back to your breath.

Keeping your mind focused on your breath, notice the part of you that is aware of your mind focusing on your breath. This awareness is a different experience and sensation than your mind's experience of breathing in and out. This awareness takes you into matrix consciousness.

Focus on this sensation of awareness. Feel how this awareness permeates your whole body. Follow this awareness into the coherent fluid medium in the tubules. Notice how this awareness is coherent throughout your microfibrils and microtubules. Stay focused on your coherent awareness. As your brain consciousness shifts away into thought. Gently bring it back to focus on your breath.

Continue to keep your mind focused on your breath while you experience awareness, consciousness and coherence in your microfibrils and microtubules.

Let go of your focus on your breath, and let the conscious awareness in your microfibrils and microtubules engage in experiencing the external world. Come back to your breath.

Return to stillness and notice the different sensations in the body.

ENLIVENING THE INTERNAL MATRIX

I have introduced the reader in this book to the amazing, interconnected, coherent nature of the microfibril/organized water matrix of the fascia. We have seen that the tensegrity structure of this matrix gives us a way to move within gravity, without being pulled by it. We have seen the different qualities of conductivity, mutability, adaptability, balanced reciprocal tension and the coherent liquid crystalline nature of the fascial matrix. We have explored these as a direct experience in our bodies and used our hands to contact and move it.

This information highway, which informs our body separate from our nervous system, is a crucial part of our coherent self. It gives us immediate, instantaneous coordination to function in our complex world. We have learned that this coherence in the matrix is the key to the consciousness of wholeness and links our cells and fascia to the "big" organism of the earth and all living things.

When we enliven our microfibril/organized water matrix, shifting the inertial patterns back into the coherent whole, we are bringing this immediate coordination and coherent relationship back to its full unity. By enhancing the functions and abilities of our fascial matrix, we are allowing the dynamic experience of awareness, the full flow of consciousness, the vitality and potency of the body, and the depth of experience to permeate our whole being. This increases our health and well-being, giving us a greater capacity to live and respond to the world, to respond (not react) to our external environment.

Now let's move on to Part II, where we will explore the resources in our body, practice moving the internal matrix and use our hands to enliven matrix consciousness.

Part II

APPLICATIONS

Including:

Resources in the Body
Self-Practice
Hands-on Practice

CHAPTER 15
RESOURCES IN THE BODY

INTRODUCTION

From the beginning of our lives, we go through many changes and patterns that are integral to our life cycle. Each pattern and change turns the wheel of evolution bringing us to our present self. As we grow and develop, earlier patterns that have been overlaid by later patterns still remain in the crystal memory structures of our bodies. These older patterns provide resources for our body, and they anchor our dynamic diversity.

As life asks us to limit our capacity to the work at hand, many of these resources are hidden and go unused. But by bringing back into consciousness some of these anchors of relationship, we enhance their influence on our capacity for adaptation, engagement, disengagement, reflection, relationship and connection.

Much of Western medicine concentrates on the defects of the organism and the diseases these defects may cause. This approach is largely myopic, as it disregards the influences of the whole organism and its own inherent resources. Western medical procedures often involve chemical and mechanical interventions that create more foreign input for our bodies to contend with. Levels of well-being and vitality go largely unconsidered, and the unique configuration of one's integrated organism is not deemed important.

Working with the liquid crystalline matrix brings us into contact with our interconnected, integrated wholeness. It uses the inherent resources of our body and contacts the unique interplay between our individual experiences. Levels of well-being, vitality, potency and adaptability are the main markers of consideration for those who work the matrix. Inputs into the system include internal movements and impulses that stimulate our organism's ability to shift and return to its balanced, coherent nature.

CONCEPTS IN WESTERN MEDICINE	CONCEPTS IN MOVING THE INTERNAL MATRIX
• New disease	• Dynamic Wholeness
• Invasive, toxic treatment	• Reconnect Inertial Patterns
• Separate disease forms	• Enliven and open inertial patterns
• Naming of defect	• Inertial patterns
• Individual symptoms	• Repetitive patterns
• Separation of parts	• Integrated system
• Mechanical body	• Dynamic, potent organism

In this part of the book we look at our different resources and use Explorations to enhance these resources. By bringing these resources into consciousness and using them during appropriate challenges in life, we can bring the full capacity of our organism into play and broaden the repetitive, limiting way we live in this world.

The resources we will look at include stems cells and the mesodermic field, the midline and primitive streak, heart coherence and the SA node, the holographic, fractal nature of quantum coherence, the automatic shifting fulcrums that create balanced reciprocal tensions, and the self-recognition of our signature wave pattern. These resources help us choose how to relate to the external and internal inputs from our environment. These are resources we can use to support inherent health, inherent vitality and inherent balance.

CHAPTER 16
STEM CELLS AND MESODERMIC FIELD MEMORY

From the time of the fertilized egg, until the body unfolds in the pushing and pulling and shaping of the fetus, the cells that are reproducing are our stem cells. Stem cells are "pleuripotent," meaning that they can differentiate and develop into different cells determined by the function they need to perform. All stem cells have the same genetic code in their DNA, but retain the potential to become any cell type.

A fertilized egg soon divides into two layers, and these layers hold two different types of stem cells that readying themselves for the different jobs they will perform. Then, once the primitive streak moves between the two layers of the embryo and creates the mesoderm, the three resultant layers of stem cells are the ingredients needed to create a diverse, dynamic organism.

Once our body is formed in utero, most of our stem cells have become function-specific cells, creating organs, tissue systems and connective tissue. However, some stem cells continue to exist throughout our bodies. There are stem cells in our bone marrow, still with the potency to be different types of blood cells. There are also stem cells in our fascia, muscle, bone, fat, organs and brain tissue that are still undifferentiated into any specialized cell. As we age, our stem cell potency is reduced.

Once a stem cell has become specialized it loses its ability to develop into other cell types, and it has "brakes" that prevent it from expressing its stem cell origins. However, all cells have a memory of stem cell expression and "know" their origin in the embryonic field. They also are influenced by the environment (epigenetics) and can change expression in response to both internal and external inputs.

Stem cells are the expression of our adaptable, changeable, malleable capacity to live in this world. Their field and energy potency gives us the ability to redefine, redirect and recalibrate our internal and external relationships.

This memory of infinite possibility in our functional cells, as well as in our adult stem cells, helps us to begin again, dissolving our fixed identities, bringing us into the present moment of discovery. This ability to recall the potency of the undifferentiated stem cells in our body is a valuable resource in adapting to our environment. Using this potent stem cell energy—to open the possibilities in the system and to give it the ability to reestablish its original design—is crucial to living in this complex and increasingly toxic world.

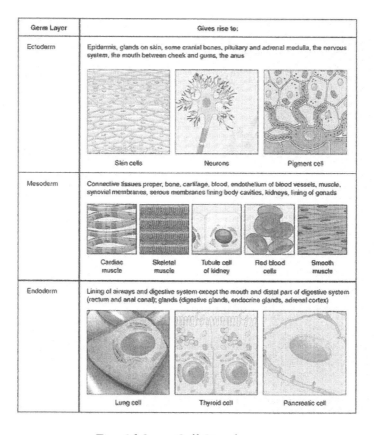

Fig. 56 Stem Cell Development

EXPLORATION 56: FINDING YOUR STEM CELL POTENCY

Find a comfortable place to lie down and settle into your body. Let your awareness move to the cellular level of your body. Imagine all of the different cells in the body with their semipermeable membranes and cytoskeletons of microtubules. Notice how the cells are pressed together within a fluid medium. Notice how the cells are moving and shifting, rippling with relationship inside and outside. Follow the similar cell groups that form your bones, muscles, organs and fascial matrix.

Bring your awareness to the cells of the fascial matrix. Imagine you can roll back time and watch, like a movie running backwards, your cells as they un-divide into the cells that existed first, all the way back to their roots as stem cells. Go all the to the embryo. Notice the disc of two layers. Then as it attaches to the mother, watch the primitive streak pulse between them and form a third layer. Watch the stem cells in this third layer (mesoderm) pulsate between the other two (ectoderm and endoderm) stem cell layers. Feel the potency of the mesodermic stem cells. Feel how they are waiting to feel the push and pull of becoming. Feel how they are waiting to be called to function within the fascial matrix.

Now roll forward in time and imagine the mesodermic cells creating the internal matrix, building, shaping and forming spaces for the other stem cells to fill. Imagine that as these stem cells become connective tissues they begin to form the bones, ligaments, tendons and muscles within the spaces the matrix is creating. Notice that some stem cells reproduce and become a specific cell type, while other stem cells remain as stem cells, keeping their potency.

Bring your awareness to your present cells. Scan through your cells and find the stem cells that are still in the mix of functional cells. Feel their potency within the tissues and layers of functioning systems. Let your awareness come back to your body and notice the potency you felt during the Exploration.

EMBRYONIC FIELD POTENTIAL

The amazing journey of a fertilized egg into a new born baby is the journey of embryology. This ability to manifest a living, growing, adapting being comes from the laws of nature, which maintain the generalized structure from which we live. Each of the different stages of development inside and outside the womb is geared towards the functional needs of the organism. These stages continue to express themselves throughout our lives, shifting from development to repair, growth to stability, and differentiation to adaptation.

Bonnie Gintis, DO: "Healing and change in an adult are guided by the same physiologic principles as growth and development of an embryo into a child…. There is a field of embryonic potential, an undifferentiated state that unfolds and guides growth and development, as well as adaptation, change and the healing process of adults."

–From *Engaging the Movement of Life: Exploring Health and Embodiment Through Osteopathy and Continuum*, **North Atlantic Books, pg. 118.**

This consistency in embryonic knowledge and wisdom is embedded in the tissues of our body through the embryonic field. It influences all the ways in which we live, create, move, change, adapt and grow in life. It is an amazing resource and influence on our bodies. With its direct relationship to the forces of the internal and external environments, the embryonic field guides our tissues' relationships throughout our life on the planet. To invoke its wisdom as we move and adapt in life can bring clarity, efficiency and potency to the changes being asked of us in life.

MESENCHYME

Mesenchyme is the watery, potentized matrix that is part of our stem cells' environment, giving a medium for the forces of development and differentiation to occur. It holds the space for the pulsation of life to evolve through the phases of embryonic development. All of our connective tissues, along with the notochord, cranial base and meninges are derived from mesenchyme. It is an amazing source of potency that has the capacity to become many different tissues through the forces of gravity and the push/pull of cell division. It is another resource in the body's embryological field of potential.

Charles Ridley: "Mesenchyme... is the template in which the force of primary respirations combines with levity and gravity to create all bodily functions, including sentience."

–From *Stillness: Biodynamic Cranial Practice and the Evolution of Consciousness*, North Atlantic Books, pg. 200.

MESODERMIC FIELD MEMORY

The mesodermic field is the gathering of the unique qualities that shape and form the connective tissues of our body. It is the field of potency emanating from the stem cells and mesenchyme fluid matrix. It includes the qualities of our primitive streak or first impulse of life, our ability to move and invite functional direction, our ability to shift and change to meet functional needs of the bigger organism, and our ability to be a communication network for the bigger organism.

These qualities of mutability, adaptability and functional orientation are held in the cell memory of all of our mesodermic tissues, including the fascia. These qualities give our body the support it needs to survive in our ever-changing world. This field memory is a great resource for our body, giving us the ability to be present and engaged in our life.

Bonnie Gintis, DO: "The mutability of tissues derived from this (mesodermic) embryonic layer of cells is inherent in their nature… No other cells in the body change as quickly and easily, or move as freely through the body, as those derived from this layer."

–From *Engaging the Movement of Life: Exploring Health and Embodiment Through Osteopathy and Continuum,* North Atlantic Books, pg. 156.

EXPLORATION 57: FINDING YOUR MUTABLE MESODERMIC LAYERS

Find a comfortable place to lie down and settle into your body. Bring your awareness to your internal matrix. Feel the layers of cells, microfibrils and organized water that make up your internal matrix. Notice that these same ingredients form your tendons, ligaments, muscles and bones, interconnecting your whole connective tissue mesodermic system. Feel the interconnected flow between your connective tissues. Notice the wave patterns rippling through the organized water in your matrix.

Let your body begin to glide gently and move your connective tissues. Feel how they shift and change to the inputs of push/pull and gravity. Feel how they adapt and change to the inputs while continuing to stay connected. Feel how they communicate and exchange information. Feel how they support and hold the spaces for the nerves, organs and gut tube. Notice how the mesodermic layers of connective tissue feel different than the ectodermic layers of sensory and motor nerves or the endodermic layers of the digestive tract. Notice how the mesodermic layers connect throughout your body, while your other layers have specific pathways they follow.

Come back to stillness and notice the felt sense of your mesodermic connective tissue layers in contrast to your ectodermic and endodermic layers.

CHAPTER 17
THE PRIMITIVE STREAK AND MIDLINE

The primitive streak—the first impulse or movement we make—starts the dance of creating our bodies out of the embryo. At day 14 in the embryo's development, when the bilaminal disc of endoderm and ectoderm attaches to the uterus, a wave of nourishment comes between the two layers of stem cells. This wave is the primitive streak that begins to organize our cells into a human being. Our primitive streak creates a third layer called the mesoderm, which will become the midline of the body.

Our embryos use the primitive streak pulsation to understand left/right orientation, gravity and our body's reciprocal tension balance. As we recall this first pulsation in the body, we can find our way to the midline. Midline is the place of neutral, the place from which our life first differentiated and became a complex organism. As a cellular memory, it returns our body to the place of beginning, before patterning and identity began. The midline reconnects us to our beginnings and helps orient our cells to gravity. Our primitive streak memory can be a great resource for us, helping us to let go of dominant patterning and rebalance left and right.

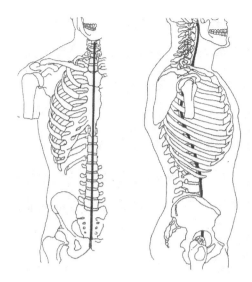

Fig. 57 Midline in adult

THE THREE MIDLINES

Three midlines are created from our three stem cell layers, representing the functional/structural divisions of the body. Each midline is connected through its stem cell layer and creates the midline and focal point for those organs involved.

The ectoderm layer of stem cells forms our central nervous system, peripheral epidermis and sensory neurons, as well as sebaceous, mammary and lacrimal glands. This network of communication and response is vital for the functioning of our organism. The midline for this layer is the space where the cerebrospinal fluid lives, that is, the inner chambers of our spine.

The mesoderm layer of cells comes from the primitive streak and forms through the notochord, which becomes the bones of the vertebra, the fascia, muscles, etc. It also creates our urinary and reproductive structures, as well as our heart, blood and blood vessels. The midline for this layer is anterior to the spine, and it is the one we work with in this book to recalibrate our fascial matrix.

The endoderm layer of stem cells forms the gut tube and the linings of our hollow vessels, including our lungs, larynx, trachea and bronchi. It creates the most anterior midline that connects with the whole digestive and respiratory systems, taking in nourishment and discarding waste.

THE MESODERMIC MIDLINE

The mesodermic midline—which is neither left/right, or anterior/posterior, but is truly in the middle of our body—lies in front (anterior) to our spine. You can trace it down the middle line of your cranium, through the middle of your sphenoid bone, behind your trachea and esophagus, in front of your spinal vertebrae, along the anterior midline of your sacrum, to the tip of your coccyx. At the third ventricle in the cranium and the coccyx, your three midlines come together and terminate. These are potent points along the midline.

Your midline is more than simply the space it represents. It is the place of stillness and neutral, where your body comes to pause and recalibrate. It is the fulcrum that our resonance and conduction spiral around, creating our own bioelectric field of verticality for communication with the earth and sky. It is the core and center of our integrated body, and an important resource that can regenerate, enliven and recalibrate our body's integrated energy and information exchange. It is a focal point for healing, awareness, consciousness and regeneration.

Charles Ridley: "The midline is a vertical line of stillness with a bioelectric field that is a potent reference beam around which the holographic matrix orders all function and structure during embryonic generation, maintenance, healing, perception, and the evolution of consciousness."

–From *Stillness: Biodynamic Cranial Practice and the Evolution of Consciousness*, North Atlantic Books, pg. 202.

EXPLORATION 58: FINDING YOUR MESODERMIC MIDLINE

Find a comfortable place to sit with your feet on the ground and spine aligned. Settle into your body. Feel your way through your layers of tissue until you come to the middle of your torso, head and sacrum.

Imagine a line from the top of your head through the sphenoid bone behind your eyes, down the front of your spine and sacrum, to the tip of your coccyx. Bring your awareness to this line, your midline, and feel the sense of neutral, where stillness and lack of push and pull are found. Continue through the midline of your legs to the bottom of your feet and into the ground. Hold your focus on your whole midline.

Feel your tissues begin to organize around your midline. Feel your tissues increase their coherence as they relate to your midline.

Notice the movements and stillness, the ebb and flow emanating from your midline. Bring your attention to the left and right sides of your body and feel the tug of gravity. Return your awareness to the midline, then back out to the sides of the body, feeling their differences and their relationship.

Stand up and move slowly while maintaining your awareness at your midline.

We use the midline to bring our energies and thoughts to a still, silent place. From this place of neutral we can engage in the self-practice of moving our internal matrix, or work with others. We can access the midline to create calmness and spaciousness, dissolving the worries and distressed voices within us. We can focus on the midline to reenergize and heal old traumas. Furthermore, we can use the midline to disrupt old patterns that create imbalances left to right, limit range of motion, and reduce our movement capacity.

We use the midline to integrate our matrix after hands-on work or self-practice. We contact our midline to ground and stabilize ourselves when moving from one activity to another. The midline becomes our place fro, which we relation to gravity, the people we touch and the environment we live in.

Once you are familiar with finding your mesodermic midline and maintaining the sensation of it in your body, you can use it whenever you need support in your daily life.

CHAPTER 18
HEART RESONANCE AND COHERENCE

HEART RESONANCE

Our heart's resonance originates from the splanchnic mesoderm in the primitive streak, which are clustering cells that conduct an electromagnetic field. This field becomes the pulsation which moves our blood through the developing embryo until our heart is formed. These pacemaker cells entrain all of our developing cells and resonate our integrated electromagnetic field from the core of our midline out into the environment. Once our heart is formed these pacemaker cells settle near the center of our body, continuing to be the conductor of our signature resonance.

Our heart's resonance harmonizes with the other oscillations in our body to create our signature wave pattern. When these oscillations come together in a holographic, coherent rhythm, the vitality and potency of our body is maintained. This powerfully integrated electromagnetic field of our heart is a fractal resonance of the electromagnetic pulsating field in our cells and in our fascia.

HEART COHERENCE

The fractal resonance that pulsates through the microtubules in our cells, the microfibril/organized water of our fascia matrix, our heart, and our glial cells in the brain… all of these create a strong electromagnetic field that protects, coheres and self-reflects on our living being. When these components are in harmony internally and externally, they create heart coherence within our resonant body.

With every external and internal input that our body engages in, our heart resonance responds accordingly, exchanging the information through our fractal matrices. Some inputs, including emotional, physiological or environmental disharmony, change our heart's rhythmic field, impacting our pacemaker cells, which are called the sinoatrial node.

Charles Ridley: "Each change in the body — or in any signal from the environment — impacts the cardiac cycle, altering the heart's electromagnetic field in an ever changing wave display that has no measurable end. The electromagnetic field of the heart emits a torus-shape fractal pattern (an infinite, nonlinear, multidimensional, lemniscate figure-eight pattern) that continually reorients to an ever-shifting fulcrum."

–From *Stillness: Biodynamic Cranial Practice and the Evolution of Consciousness*, **North Atlantic Books, pg. 189.**

SINOATRIAL NODE

The sinoatrial node (SA node) is the cluster of pacemaker cells in our heart that begins as the resonator of the electromagnetic field of our body and becomes the pacemaker (or rhythm maker) of our heartbeat. These cells are very sensitive to internal and external inputs, and they have a direct connection to the limbic system (emotional center) of our brain. They continue to pulsate the electromagnetic field of our body, as well as determine the rhythm and response of our heart field.

This electromagnetic field that emanates from the SA node of our heart pulsates through our microtubules and microfibrils. By focusing on this fulcrum and harmonizing the inputs to it, we can use the SA node as a resource to enliven and cohere the electromagnetic fields in our microtubules and microfibrils.

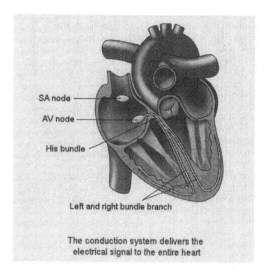

SA node

AV node

His bundle

Left and right bundle branch

The conduction system delivers the
electrical signal to the entire heart

Fig. 58 Sino Atrial Node

EXPLORATION 59: FINDING YOUR SA NODE

Find a comfortable place to sit with your feet on the ground. Settle into your body. Let your breath calm and slow your body down. Feel the letting go and relaxing as you breathe slowly.

Focus your awareness to the left of your sternum, where your heart lives. Let your hands touch the area and connect with the vibration coming out of your heart. Breathe into the area and enhance the vibration. Feel the rhythm of your heart slow.

Let your awareness move to the top of your heart. Notice the cluster of cells at your right atria. Feel how they hold a coherent charge that pulls them together. Feel the vibration that comes from that cluster of cells. Feel the vibration move out in a sphere that surrounds your body.

Feel the vibration in your microfibril/organized water matrix and how it includes the vibration coming out of your SA Node. Feel the potency of your resonance. Connect with your signature resonance.

Take your hands off your heart and let your breath bring you back into the boundaries of your body. Feel how this boundary has changed.

EXPLORATION 60: FINDING YOUR HEART COHERENCE

Find a comfortable place to lie down and settle into your body. Let your breath relax you. With each exhale let yourself relax even more, moving your awareness into the body's vibrational patterns.

Move your attention to your heart, to the left of your sternum. Feel its physical boundaries as well as its vibrational boundaries. Let your awareness follow the rippling of coherent energy that moves ftrom your heart center out and back, filling you and the space around you with the vibration of your heart beating.

Now bring your awareness to your SA node cells. Feel the pull between these cells and follow the vibration as it moves through your body. Notice how the microfibril/organized water matrix of your fascia is also moving the vibration of these electric cells.

Now feel the connections between these two vibrations of heart center and SA node. Notice the strength and potency of the two vibrations as they move throughout your body and the space around. Feel the protection and wholeness in their connection.

Now let go of the coherence and let your breath take you into a deeper relaxation. Notice how the boundaries of the body have changed.

CHAPTER 19
INHERENT HEALTH

TO BE ALIVE

Our body is an incredible, self-sustaining, self-supporting, self-regulating organism. Its ability to maintain all of our complex functions independently while shifting and changing to the inputs and work of being alive gives it the capacity to maintain health, vitality and balance.

This complexity of action, interaction and energy availability is supported and regulated by the immediate exchange of information in our microfibril/organized water matrix, in community with our nervous system and the chemical reactions in our tissues.

We can enliven our body, enhancing it abilities to self-regulate and maintain its homeostasis, by complexifying and integrating the microfibrils in our fascial matrix, returning them to their original state of mutable, mobile, movement efficiency. This keeps our body informed of the infinite numbers of weak signals, strong signals and inputs it must respond to.

SELF-SUSTAINING, SELF-REGULATING, SELF-SUPPORTING SYSTEM

Our bodies are self-sustaining and self-regulating systems that can listen to the information coming through our microfibril/organized water matrix and respond immediately through the appropriate tissues and chemical interactions. This ability to sustain and regulate our functions allows us to move and live in the world without the awareness of this process. When we tap into the awareness of this conductive, coherent, self-regulating capacity, we tap into the inherent health of the body.

EXPLORATION 61: ENGAGING THE SELF-REGULATING SYSTEM

Find a comfortable place to lie down and settle into your body. Begin by focusing on the outside of your skin. Bring your awareness to its ability to take information from the outside environment and communicate it into your body. Imagine the microtubules in your cells and your microfibril/organized water matrix reaching out to your skin, taking in the information and informing the rest of your body through its conductive matrix.

Move your awareness to the blood-side of your skin and your superficial matrix. Feel how your microfibrils vibrate and move information throughout the layers of your matrix. Let your focus widen to your awareness of the self-regulating, continually shifting, adapting system within your body. Feel the massively complex exchange that is happening in your matrix. Feel the coherence in this exchange.

Allow your internal awareness of the microfibril/organized water matrix to find a place where an inertial pattern has been created. Let the enlivened matrix engage with this inertial pattern in your matrix. Pause, and let your inertial pattern dissolve and reconnect to the whole matrix through your body's drive to optimal health.

Feel the exchange of information as well as the sustaining continuance of your signature vibration. Allow your awareness to feel the wholeness of your system and notice the places of exchange at each connection along your microfibrils.

Take a moment to feel amazement and gratitude for your self-regulating system.

Charles Ridley: "The self-regulatory system is the matrix—the liquid ground substance—that outwardly bathes and resides within all cells, providing the means for global body-wide communication, interconnectivity, coherent perception, and response. The self-regulatory system communicates quantum vibratory information throughout the whole body simultaneously and at the speed of light (or faster) through the process of coherence."

–From *Stillness: Biodynamic Cranial Practice and the Evolution of Consciousness*, North Atlantic Books, pg. 209.

INHERENT HEALTH

Our bodies are geared to self-heal and balance as we move through life. They are designed to maintain steady levels of energy, focus, awareness and consciousness. Our body is innately moving back to the place of optimal health. Its response to the external and internal signals it receives is supported by the crystal memory of our embryological journey. We are wired to return to the optimal level of health and vitality as we move, grow, develop and function.

Bonnie Gintis, DO: "The Health is an aspect of life that has expression as long as a person is alive, regardless of the presence of disease, dysfunction or injury. The Health has no opposite. It is unequivocally complete and present as long as there is life…Unlike Health, wellness can be altered, diseased, diminished, deranged, or become inertial."

–From *Engaging the Movement of Life: Exploring Health and Embodiment Through Osteopathy and Continuum*, North Atlantic Books, pgs. 131-132.

INHERENT VITALITY AND BALANCE

The vitality and balance that informs the health of our organism is determined by the movement cycles in our body. Whether is it the physical movement, where the balanced reciprocal tension of our biotensegrity returns to balance when it is pushed and pulled, or the microscopic conductive rhythms that shift and change our bioelectric matrix, the moving rhythms and cycles allow us to filter through the inputs without permanent change. When we are engaged in the moving, changing, shifting cycles of nature, within and without, we are truly in the larger field of relationship of the big organism (which includes all of the living systems of the Earth).

EXPLORATION 62: ENGAGING THE INHERENT HEALTH

Find a comfortable place to lie down and settle into your body. Let your awareness focus on your breath, heart beat and slower rhythms, feeling the cycles that they bring to the vibrational patterns in your matrix.

Feel your body's consistent, moving pattern of input, exchange and adaptation. Settle into this internal movement. Notice the fascial matrix that moves your vibrational pattern, the exchange that happens in your cell membranes, and the shifting that happens in the chemistry, reciprocal tension and functioning of your tissues. Feel the ability of your system to self-correct, self-organize and adapt to inputs in the system.

Now focus on the external environment. Feel how the external inputs in the environment move through your skin and microfibril/organized water matrix, informing the cells of your body. Notice how your system shifts and adapts to these inputs.

Now that you have felt the engaging system, move beneath it to your body's *awareness* of this moving system. Feel the confidence and coherence. Feel the vitality and balance underneath this rhythm. Take a moment to be informed by your inherent health, as well as the balance that maintains awareness of your natural rhythms and your relationship to the surrounding world. Smile into your inherent health, feeling gratitude for its ability to be consistent in the changing medium of life.

Come back into stillness and feel the vitality of your whole being.

CHAPTER 20
SELF-RECOGNITION

CELL RECOGNITION

Our cells, as well as our conscious being, recognize us through the boundaries and multiple markers of identity. Our cell membrane has many surface markers that identify what is related to us and what is not... a sort of lock and key system. Our immune cells have ways to identify those cells that are a part of us and those that are not. Our vibrational wave pattern brings coherence to our cells within the ever-changing internal environment of our body. Our vibrational wave pattern is recognized by all the cells in our body.

Sondra Barrett, Ph.D.: "Although it is well established that physical markings, shape and touch are essential in enabling cells to recognize other cells and molecules, some scientists are now theorizing that molecular vibrations also play a part in recognition."

–From *Secrets of Your Cells: Discovering Your Body's Inner Intelligence*, Sounds True, pg. 29.

COMPLEXITY OF PATTERNS IN THE FIELD

The vibrational wave pattern of our body is unique and complex, holding all of the rhythms that pulse through our systems. This complexity pulls together a coherent conductive pattern that is recognized by every cell in our body. This coherent pattern conducts fractally through our cells, fascia and out into our heart field. As our unique vibrational wave pattern moves through our bioelectric matrix, it does not disturb the individual wave patterns of breath, heartbeat, fluid tides and movement in our body. This ability to have independent and interdependent rhythms in our body allows us to have separate functions within our integrated whole.

ENTANGLED RHYTHMS

These complex wave patterns interact in the field as they move through our cells, tissues and the microfibrils in our fascia. As they interact, they become entangled and become our signature signal. This entangled quantum wave continues to shift and change as our experiences and inputs add more wave patterns. This entangled wave is the movement of consciousness.

———————

Mae-Wan Ho, Ph.D.: "The 'wave function' of consciousness never collapses (c.f. Schommers), but is always changing, and always unique as it is "coloured" by all the tones of our personality and experience. Each significant experience becomes entangled in our being, constituting new wave function, in much the same way that particles of independent origins become entangled after they interacted."

–From *The Rainbow and the Worm: The Physics of Organisms*, World Scientific, *pg. 333.*

———————

SIGNATURE WAVE

The signature wave that pulsates through the conductive fields in our body can be felt by ourselves as well as others. Have you ever walked into a room and sensed another person and felt their signature wave? We usually take that sensation and let the mind judge and discern its compatibility with our own signature wave.

This is another way we recognize ourselves in contrast to others.

EXPLORATION 63: SENSING OUR ENTANGLED SIGNATURE WAVE

Find a comfortable place to lie down and settle into your body. Begin by tracking your breath, noticing the breath wave pattern that moves through your microfibril/ organized water matrix. As you draw your awareness to your breath wave pattern, notice it coming to the foreground as an individual wave.

Continue by tracking your heartbeat wave pattern, your cranial wave pattern, your midline wave pattern and your full body wave pattern. Notice that you can track each wave pattern individually throughout your fascial matrix.

Now let your awareness draw those rhythms together as they move through your fascial matrix, and feel the entangled signature wave that they create. Feel the depth and fullness of your signature wave. Feel how it pulsates through your skin and out into the world.

Let your focus soften and notice other wave patterns entangling into this wave. Notice other wave patterns that come from your mind, memory and external stimulus. Notice how these wave patterns subside when your focus moves to another.

Bring your focus back to stillness and notice the different sensations in your body.

CHAPTER 21
RESPONSIVE SHIFTING FULCRUMS

BALANCED RECIPROCAL TENSION

Our body is in constant movement, from the atomic level of protons and electrons to its physical engagement through space. These movements are articulated through the changing fulcrums of tensile and compression forces. In order for our body to maintain independent and interdependent activities, it must engage in a balancing of these reciprocal tensions in its fractal biotensegrity matrix in order to create stability and flexibility. We are never in a state of fully balanced reciprocal tension, since we are constantly shifting our relationships to gravity, push and pull forces and inertial patterns. This dynamic, reciprocal relationship of suspension and compression is a constant dance in the world we live in; when we touch into this balancing tension matrix, we can feel the buoyancy and spaciousness of the body.

FULCRUMS

The fulcrums in the middle of the reciprocal tension are places of stillness, while the bioelectric matrix moves and shifts around them. These fulcrums change with movement and shift in response to the forces of gravity, as we respond and flow with the movement of life. Inviting ourselves into the fulcrums' world (instead of the moving matrix world) allows us to feel that moment of stillness and center. The main fulcrum for our whole body is the midline.

Inertial patterns in our body have their own semi-permanent fulcrums that our resonance circles and flows around. These inertial fulcrums are constantly drawing energy through friction and redirection, competing with the flow in the whole organism.

EXPLORATION 64: FINDING THE FULCRUM LEVEL OF STILLNESS

Find a comfortable place to lie down and settle into your body. Focus on your internal matrix. Feel your layers of microfibrils and their internal engagement.

Allow your microfibril/organized water matrix to move gently and slowly your body. As your body shifts its reciprocal tension to move within and through space, notice the fulcrum around that reciprocal tension. As your body spirals and rotates, notice the fulcrum at the center of your movement. Notice how your body is shifting its relationship to gravity. Notice the fulcrum that your body moves around.

Continue to let your internal matrix move you slowly and gently. Turn your focus to the fulcrum at the center of your movement instead of at the level of your microfibrils shifting and changing.

Hold your focus on the fulcrum as you move, and notice its contrasting stillness to the moving parts. Notice how, as you change direction, your fulcrum also changes. Keep your focus on that fulcrum. There may be more than one fulcrum as you move your limbs and torso.

Come back to stillness and bring your awareness to your midline. Feel its level of stillness and its relationship to the reciprocal tension in the whole body. Notice the different sensations in the body.

RESPONSIVE SHIFTING FULCRUMS

The responsive shifting fulcrums in our body — whether at the microtubule cellular level, the microfibril level or the collagen web level — are the fulcrums that arise when force, wave pulsation or movement create a pull or push on our body, bringing shifts in matrix configuration. Because we are always in a state of movement, no matter how minute, this shifting is continual. The healthy body is constantly able to respond by shifting the fulcrums around such movement while maintaining an overall balanced, coherent, buoyant space.

This ability to shift the fulcrum and let the matrix dance around it is a great resource and asset for our gravity-oriented body. By allowing our body and consciousness to connect with the stillness of the fulcrum, as well as to move with the constantly rebalancing matrix, we can experience our dynamic, responsive, enlivened living system.

As the fulcrum shifts, it sends a stillness point back and forth from macro- to micro-levels, creating a fractal flow throughout the systems.

ALIGNMENT

When we are structurally oriented to the vertical force of gravity, we tend to look at alignment as a stationary relationship between plumb lines and three-dimensional planes. This static view negates the dynamic, moving, interrelated levels of the organism. When we see alignment as the moving quality of shifting fulcrums, we can understand the stability and flow of the systems.

Bonnie Gintis, DO: "There is no such thing as proper alignment. Alignment is a static quality, and the body is a dynamic unit of function… If every part of the body were free to move the way it was designed to, the alignment would take care of itself."

–From *Engaging the Movement of Life: Exploring Health and Embodiment Through Osteopathy and Continuum,* **North Atlantic Books, pg. 216.**

EXPLORATION 65: MOVING FROM SHIFTING MATRIX TO SHIFTING FULCRUM

Find a comfortable place to lie down and settle into your body. Focus on your internal matrix. Feel its fulcrum at the midline and the reciprocal tension around it.

Let your internal matrix initiate movement gently and slowly. Focus on the reciprocal tension as it shifts and changes with your movement. Notice how the microfibrils in your matrix shift their relationship to each other, maintaining the reciprocal tension. Let your awareness stay in the shifting matrix, feeling how your body shifts with the movement so that your alignment and relationship to gravity are maintained.

Come back to stillness and focus on your midline fulcrum. Let your internal matrix initiate movement, and keep your focus on the fulcrum at the center of that movement. Follow the fulcrum as it changes with each change in movement. Allow your awareness to stay in the stillness at the center of your movements, as your body shifts and changes its microfibril connections.

As you continue to move from your internal matrix, move your awareness back and forth between your shifting matrix and your shifting fulcrum.

Come back to stillness. Keep your awareness on your midline fulcrum and notice the different sensations in your body.

CHAPTER 22
SELF-PRACTICE

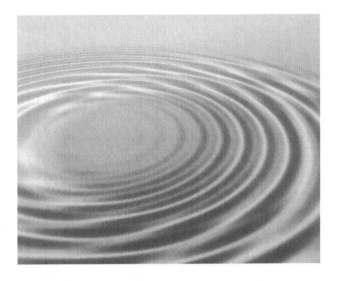

We can enliven our internal matrix by exploring its multidirectional gliding, waving and spiral movements, opening and suspending our fascial web as we invite our microfibrils to shift and change. When we move our fascial system in these ways, we warm the tissue from gel to sol, complexifying the crystal-line matrix and restoring the balance between tensile and compressive forces.

The method by which we can accomplish all of this is called *self-practice*, which can have a wide variety of benefits. By exploring and moving our lay-ers of fascial webbing, we can find places of density and inertia, then use our movements to return the matrix to its original, spongy, buoyant self. We move within the space of our bodies, using slow micro-movements that open into flowing movements from head to toe. As we change shape, density and matrix configurations, the internal systems of our bodies are nourished, supported and interconnected.

We will connect to the conductive nature of the fascia by focusing on the pulsations and rhythmic waves that move through our body. By varying pulsation, or creating a new impulse, we can activate our bioelectric matrix, enlivening the conductive capacity of our fascial tissue. These internal movements and patterns are not initiated by our sensory/motor neurological patterning and have a great potential to shift our focus of movement from levering and moving through space to the pulsating of the primal rhythms of life within us.

This self-discovery engages our awareness to the pulsations that move along the microfibril/organized water pathways, and to their dance of spiraling, connecting and moving. When we move internally we touch all the microtubules in the cells and all the microfibrils in our connective tissues, because our system is constantly in relationship, both fractally and through the coherence in the conductive pathway. We can sense our individuality internally, and we can feel the interconnectedness to the external environment and the biosphere surrounding us.

During self-practice, we shift from engaging our sensory/motor, input/movement response to engaging in the rippling pulsation of our ever-adapting fascial matrix. This wave movement is activated by changes in the microfibril connections that shift the organized water conductive pathways in our matrix. By enlivening this moving, spiraling, adapting matrix, we build an internal ability to adapt to the pressures, traumas and habitual nature of our being.

Self-practice has a basic sequence. To begin, we warm the fascial web, then move the tissue in multidirectional ways, move the fascial sleeve, use micro-movements around the spine, and give the tissue the ability to move freely, unwinding and recalibrating. This basic sequence is used in the beginning of each Exploration, before we focus on different aspect of the enlivened tissue.

Below are five different Explorations that will focus on variance of pulsation, streaming from the midline, fulcrums, mobility and motility, suspension and coherence, specific layers of the matrix, and inertial patterns. Each Exploration uses the basic sequence described above to create a felt sense of each quality of fascia, and specific ways to emphasize their enlivenment.

We will start with a list of concepts that guide the movement exploration. Remember to use these directives as you begin to enliven your internal matrix.

CONCEPTS TO REMEMBER WHEN ENGAGING THE FASCIAL LIQUID CRYSTALLINE MATRIX

- Move within the space of your body,
- instead of through the space around you.
- Notice the felt sense of your body before
- and after you glide, move and spiral.
- Take up the slack in the fascia to create a tautness
- to activate movement in the microfibrils.
- Use micro-movements
- within the microscopic layers of microfibrils.
- Use slow, flowing, gliding movements, like pouring weight
- through legs, torso and arms.
- Use figure eight movements
- at spine and within joints.
- Pulsate ebbing and flowing movements
- from midline out and back.
- Feel pulling together (coherence) and
- pulling apart (suspension) within the movements.
- Feel movements rippling through layers,
- like waves moving out from a stone dropped in water
- Find fascial movement around a fulcrum,
- and find stillness within the fulcrum.
- Let movement arise from tissue, *not* mind.
- Let your fascia move you!

BASIC SEQUENCE

WARM UP: MUSCLE MOVEMENT TO FASCIAL MOVEMENT

1. Begin by moving your arms: flex and extend your forearms, feel your muscles contracting and releasing.

2. Move around the room feeling your neuromuscular systems move your skeleton through space.

3. Vary your pace, fast and slow.

4. Use as many muscles as you can to move through space, then use as few muscles as you can.

5. Notice the fulcrum at your joints and the levering your muscles use to move your bones, and notice how some muscles contract when others extend.

6. Notice the pull on your bones from your muscle tendons and the stabilizing pull from your ligaments.

7. Push and pull, stretch and move in different relationships to gravity.

8. Come back to standing and notice how your system is warmed up and ready to glide your fascia.

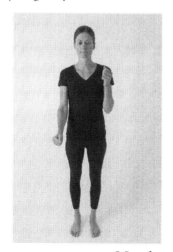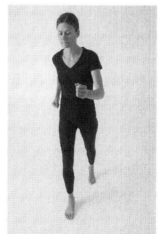

Muscle movement

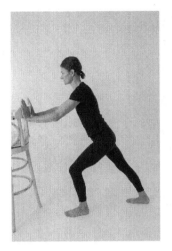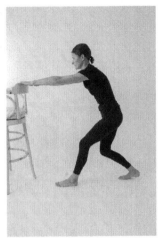

#7 Push and pull with muscles

GLIDING THE FASCIA

1. Begin on the floor, face up, legs extended and apart, arms at side. Take a minute to notice any bodily sensations as you relax.

2. Slowly pull your right heel down while your toes move up (this is called dorsiflexion of the foot), rotating around the ankle joint to create tautness in the back of your leg. Let the tautness glide slowly and gently up the back of the leg. Don't stretch; slide and glide.

3. Slowly press the toes on your right foot down while your heel moves up toward your leg (plantar flexion of the foot), feeling the pull, then glide up the front of your foot. Let the tautness glide through the front of the ankle and through the two bones in the lower leg.

4. Repeat back and forth, letting your glide move further up the leg to the hips, torso, shoulder and head. As you glide up the right side of the body, bring the head down when the toes are pointing down and let the head move up and back when the toes are pointing up. the head flex. Continue until you feel a smooth even glide up and down the right side from head to toe.

5. Repeat on the left side.

6. Bring your arms out to your sides, and slowly glide the right arm away from the torso. Start by spreading your fingertips, letting the internal movement glide through the forearm to the upper arm, to the shoulder. Then, gently glide the arm towards the torso, starting at the sternum, sliding through the ribs, shoulder, upper arm, lower arm, hands and fingertips. Repeat the glide back and forth. Repeat with left arm. Then glide back and forth from right hand to left hand.

7. Raise your arms above your head. Give a slight tautness to your left side by holding the foot as you glide slowly and gently from you left foot, upper legs, hips and torso, through your shoulder and up the left arm to the fingertips. Then create tautness in your left hand and glide back down to the left foot. You are now gliding your whole fascial sleeve from foot to fingertips, up and down the whole body. Engage the arms more by pulling to a greater tautness as you glide back and forth, increasing the amount of the fascial web you are gliding. Repeat on right side.

8. Shift to a diagonal movement from left heel to right fingertips and back. Repeat in the other direction, from right heel to left fingertips. Remember to initiate glide by holding your foot or hand, moving the sleeve until you feel a tautness. Then gradually let go of the hold at the extremity.

9. Once you have engaged your fascial sleeve in these different directions, relax and let your fascial web move on its own. Create tautness in your matrix in order to initiate glide.

10. As you feel the impulse of glide, enhance the glide and let it move throughout your body. Notice the spiraling tendencies and how you can engage more of the layers when you rotate and turn.

11. Rest, noticing the changes in your felt sense of your body.

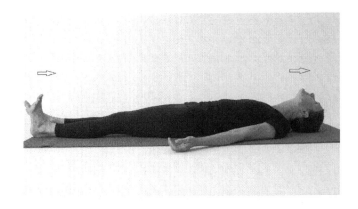

#2 Gliding the Fascia

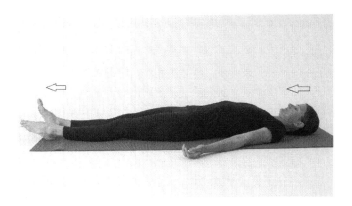

#3 Gliding the Fascia

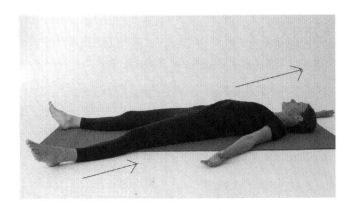

#4 Gliding the Fascia

Now we will work with some more movement exercises to vary our relationship to our internal matrix. Always be sure to perform the Basic Sequence first so that you are engaged in the internal movements of your matrix.

CHANGING RELATIONSHIP TO GRAVITY

1. Lie on your left side, bottom leg bent, top leg over bottom leg with right foot on floor.

2. Slowly move your right foot down and around the bottom leg, tracing an arc around the bottom leg. Feel the fascial matrix shifting its fulcrums to adapt to gravity.

3. Repeat on opposite side.

4. Change your relationship to gravity in other ways using a chair, pillows or props, then glide an extremity as you feel the matrix shift, continuing to complexify your fascial matrix.

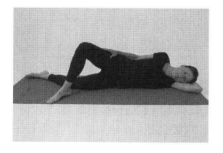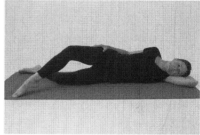
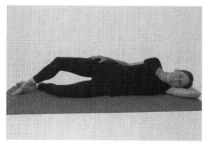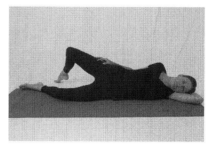

Changing your relationship to gravity

FIGURE EIGHT AROUND SPINE AND JOINTS

1. Sit in a comfortable position in a chair, with your spine aligned, your back away from the back of the chair, feet on the floor.

2. Begin by gliding back and forth slowly in a figure eight, moving from your midline out to one side, into midline and out to other side. Move the figure eight across your hips, then torso, upper back, shoulders, neck and head.

3. Starting at the top of the spinal vertebrae, do micro-movements of the figure eight back and forth between each vertebra, feeling the glide between your vertebrae and within the complex matrix between the vertebrae.

4. Let the figure eight become a flower figure, gliding around the center of your spine with the micro-movements. Let the figure eight movement become three dimensional, circling within a sphere around your spine.

5. Do micro-movements of figure eights within your ankle, knee, wrist and elbow. Let these figures eights become a flower, then a sphere.

6. Rest, noticing the change in the buoyancy around your spine and joints.

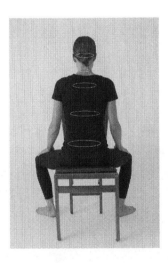

Create Figure 8 movement within circles

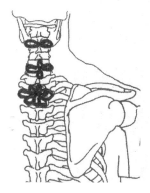

Figure 8 around spine

SPIRALING AND MOVING FASCIA

1. Lie down, arms and legs extended. Breath, relax and wait for an initiating movement from your internal matrix, then follow that movement as it glides through your fascial webbing. Let the movement glide, slowing it down if it tends to move into a faster muscle movement. If you need to start the movement with an impulse, just gently begin to rotate your leg in one direction.

2. Let your movement continue to spiral from the initial impulse until the gliding subsides and the body spreads and settles. Let another impulse engage you, following the glide of your matrix throughout your body. Let the glide twist and turn you, feeling your balanced reciprocal tension suspending you.

3. Let the movements glide slowly, noticing the ebb and flow, as well as the opening and closing. The body will tend to spiral and glide in different directions. If you keep your movements slow, you will notice your matrix shifting and changing to adapt to your relationship with gravity. Allow your movement to move slowly as far as it needs to, then feel it shift into another gliding sequence.

4. Change position on the floor, with different angles to the floor and space. Then begin a rotation and let it move you.

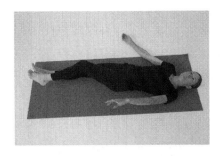
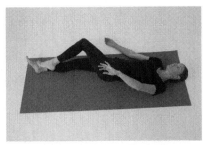
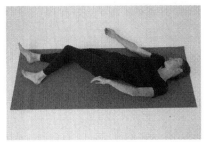
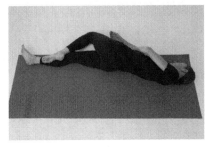

Spiraling your Fascial Matrix

Now we will concentrate on different aspects of the Basic Sequence to increase mobility, motility, suspension, coherence and complexity within microfibril/organized water matrix.

FROM GLIDE TO RESONANCE

Now that you have learned to glide, move and spiral your bioelectric matrix, your experience has recorded a felt sense of this moving structure. We will now shift our focus to the energetic field of your matrix as it pulsates wave motions through your microfibril/organized water matrix. With this new experience, you will learn to feel the streaming of wave motion, resonance and coherence in the energetic field of your matrix. These new sensations are subtle and very small. If you cannot sense them, let your imagination find them.

Again, start with the Basic Sequence (pg. 213) to enliven your fascial matrix before doing this series of Explorations.

FEELING THE PULSATIONS OF LIFE: BREATH

1. Lying on your back, focus on your breath. Feel your inhalation suspending and opening your torso space. Feel your exhalation compressing and closing that space.

2. Shift your focus to the streaming of pulsation from the center of your sternum outward as you inhale, and back to center as you exhale, like a stone being dropped in water.

3. Feel the tidal wave of pulsation as it streams out from your sternum through your torso, down your legs to your toes, down your arms to your finger tips, and up through your head. And then as it flows back to your sternum.

4. Continue to feel the waves of the stone dropped into water as you breathe, streaming out and in through your microfibril/organized water matrix.

HEARTBEAT

1. Place your hand on your heart and feel the vibrations of your heart beating.

2. Follow the pulsation of your heart as it resonates out through your torso, head and extremities.

3. Feel the pulsation as a continuous rhythm within your microfibril/organized water matrix.

CRANIAL TIDE

1. Feel the pulsation of your cranial rhythm as it rotates your matrix from a neutral position inward, pauses, then rotates your matrix outward to the neutral position. Then feel as it rotates outward from the neutral position, pauses, then rotates inward back to the neutral position.

2. Follow the ebb and flow as the cerebral spinal fluid moves towards your head and back towards your sacrum with inward and outward rotation.

MIDLINE TIDE

1. Focus on the midline in your body. Feel the pulsations streaming from your midline out to the edges of your body.

2. Feel the pulsations streaming from the edges of your body back to your midline. Feel the pulsations in the microfibril/organized water matrix.

LONGITUDINAL TIDE, EARTH TIDE

1. Focus on the bottoms of your feet and feel the pulsations from the Earth slowly streaming up your body.

2. Let the streaming resonate through the fascial matrix in your body.

3. Let the streaming move out to your hands and head. Feel the continuum of the streaming and the nourishment it provides.

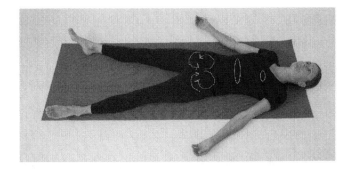

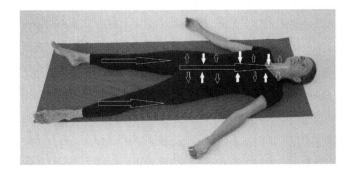

The five pulsations

INITIATING IMPULSE AND STREAMING

1. Lying on your back, arms out to your sides, start by initiating an impulse from your torso at the center of your sternum out through your right arm to the fingertips.

2. Suspend the space on the right side of your torso by gently expanding it in all directions to allow for the impulse to stream into your right arm and hand.

3. Slow the impulse down so you can feel the streaming of conduction through your microfibril/organized water matrix.

4. Let your impulse reach your fingertips by gently spreading your fingers apart. Stream the wave pattern back through your arm and torso to your sternum. Repeat, feeling the streaming like the ripples from a stone dropped in a pond, out to the edge then back.

5. Repeat the impulse from your torso out to your other arm, each leg and the top of your head.

6. Once you have completed these five different directions of impulse, notice the star-like configuration of the impulsing.

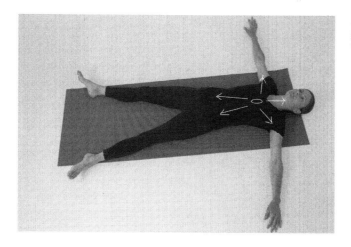

Starfish streaming

CIRCULAR PULSATION AND WAVE MOTION

1. Now start at the center of the sternum and imagine that a stone is dropped into the conductive fluid within your fascial matrix. Let the wave motion from this stone resonate out in all directions until it reaches the edges of your body.

2. Let this rippling wave motion continue from the sternum, out and then back until it is resonating throughout the fascia matrix.

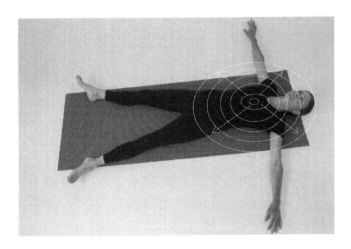

Circular pulsation

ENGAGING LAYERS WHILE GLIDING AND STREAMING

As we move our fascia, gliding and streaming through our microfibril/organized water matrix, we enliven and enhance its mutability, mobility and adaptability. The more layers of our bioelectric matrix we engage, the greater the affect. Since all of the layers are one interconnected matrix, all the moving that happens is experienced by the whole matrix. However, where we have inertial patterns or overriding compressive or tensile forces, our matrix may bypass these areas as it ripples, glides and streams. The more we shift and move our matrix by changing our relationship to gravity or using rotation to engage deeper levels, the more we engage the whole system.

GLIDING SUPERFICIAL FASCIA

1. Begin by doing steps 1-7 in **Gliding the fascia (pg. 214)** of the Basic Sequence.

2. Feel the gliding motion through the whole superficial sleeve of your fascia. Then shift your awareness to feel the wave motions streaming through your full sleeve.

Turn and rotate into deeper layers of your matrix.

1. Glide the fascia by gently and slowly rotating each extremity (hands, feet, head) in one direction, then back the other direction. Feel your matrix gliding around the other tissues until you feel it engage the matrix in your torso and hips.

2. Let the fascia of your torso, hips and other extremities engage in the gliding as your body begins to spiral and shift to engage more of your matrix. Let your whole body spiral and move.

3. Feel the streaming of wave motion through the spiral rotation as it moves into the middle layers of your matrix.

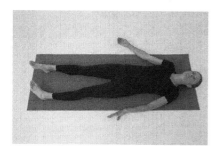
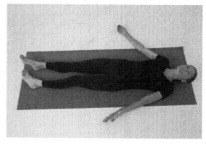
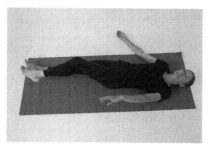
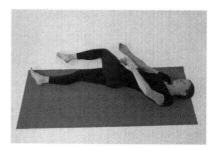

Rotating into deeper layers of Matrix

ENGAGING DEEPER LAYERS

1. Gently glide and move your internal matrix in figure eights in all directions in the pelvis, respiratory diaphragm, and shoulders.

2. Glide figure eights in all directions within the abdomen.

3. Come to stillness and let the matrix initiate movement, letting the body move in a slow, spiraling, rotating motion. Allow the movements to engage your whole body as it glides internally. Slowly glide the body within its space, as if it is pouring weight from one space to another.

4. Shift from gliding to streaming, feeling the difference between spiral, figure eight, suspending and releasing, and ebbing and flowing.

BALANCING RECIPROCAL TENSIONS

As we move, our body is continually shifting its balance with gravity in order to move with ease through space. When this balance point changes, our microfibril/organized water matrix shifts its compressive and tensile forces to restore balance. As we repeat patterns of movement, the matrix begins to form to the shifts needed in that pattern, restricting the multidirectional gliding ability of our fascia. When we experience trauma, whether physical injury or emotional distress, our microfibrils can compress and hold together (partly as memory, partly as compensation), reducing their ability to shift compressive and tensile forces. These holding patterns require significant energy, leaving us fatigued and drained. By gliding and streaming with the compressive and tensile forces, we can begin to reopen the microfibrils/organized water matrix and restore its shifting, adapting capacity.

Begin with the Basic Sequence (pg. 213) to warm and enliven the fascial matrix before exploring the compressive and tensile forces.

FINDING COMPRESSION AND TENSILE FORCES

1. Lying on your back, allow your fascia to begin to glide. The gliding movement is moving along the tensile or suspending forces of your matrix. Follow the gliding movement until it pauses.

2. When the movement pauses you have come to the compressive forces in the matrix. Pause and release all tension, letting the area spread out in all directions. Then begin to glide in a new direction. Glide with that tensile force until you meet another compressive force. Pause and spread, then glide in a new direction.

3. Let your fascia glide you through different movement sequences, feeling the tensile, suspending forces moving you to the next pause.

4. Let your matrix engage more tissue through spiraling and rotating, continuing to pause at the compressive forces, relax and spread, then glide through the tensile forces.

OPENING COMPRESSIVE HOLDING PATTERNS

1. Begin at stillness. Check into your fascial system and notice where there is tension, discomfort, any strange sensation, or a lack of sensation.

2. Focus on this place and start by using figure eight micro-movements inside it.

3. Glide away from the center of this spot until you feel the pause, then follow the matrix back to that spot. Glide away from the center at another angle and then return again to the spot. Continue to glide back and forth from the spot at different angles to create more tensile forces, spreading the compressive forces in your area of discomfort. Glide slowly and gently without increasing the discomfort or sensation.

4. Now focus on your midline fulcrum of stillness, letting it recalibrate the area you were gliding through.

5. Repeat with other areas, using tensile forces to spread out the compressed areas.

6. Finish by letting your whole matrix glide and stream as it reorganizes.

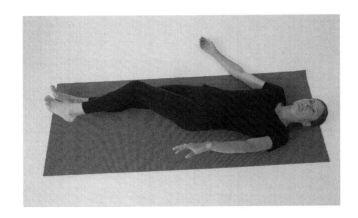

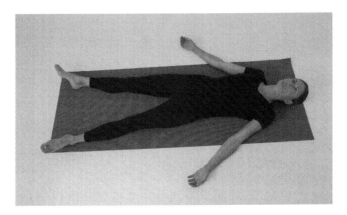

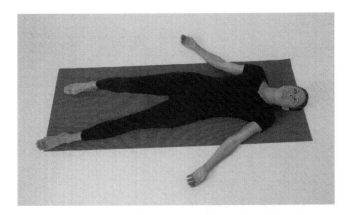

Moving with tensile and compressive forces

INERTIAL PATTERNS

Our bodies create pools and eddies of motion at areas where there is tension, compensation, past traumas, injuries or repetitive movement patterns. These separate rippling ponds are disconnected from our whole bioelectric matrix and are out of the flow of information from the conductivity within our microfibril/organized water matrix. These inertial patterns create isolated areas where deconstruction and disease can grow. By gliding them back into our integrated flow, we bring our bodies into optimal potency, vitality and well-being.

FINDING INERTIAL PATTERNS

1. Use steps 1-7 or 8&9 from Gliding the Fascia in the **Basic Sequence (pg. 213)** to bring awareness to your inertial patterns.

2. Notice the places where your glide is minimal, too fast, stops or moves around (instead of through) an area. These are indications of an inertial pattern.

3. Notice how these areas are changing as you continue to glide back and forth.

4. Adjust your assessments of the amount of glide at joints, horizontal diaphragms and boney landmarks, knowing that these areas glide differently than the longitudinal areas of arms and legs.

GLIDING THROUGH INERTIAL PATTERNS

1. Focus on an inertial patterned area. Begin by gliding your matrix outside the inertial pattern, away from the pattern and toward the pattern. Do this in all directions.

2. Use figure eight micro-movements within that inertial space.

3. Use other micro-movements such as spirals, waves and pulsations within your inertial space.

4. Initiate an impulse below your inertial pattern, gliding it through the area.

5. Initiate an impulse to the sides and above your inertial pattern, gliding through the area.

6. Glide your whole matrix from an extremity through the torso to another extremity, where the glide moves through the inertial pattern you have been working with. Notice how your inertial patterned area has changed.

STREAMING THROUGH INERTIAL PATTERNS

1. Focus on an inertial patterned area. Stream wave patterns from the outside toward the inertial pattern and away in all directions.

2. Stream wave patterns *through* your inertial patterned area.

3. Stream from your midline out through your inertial pattern and back.

FINDING DEEPER LAYERS

1. Glide around and through your inertial pattern with rotating, spiraling movements, engaging the deeper layers that may be influenced by the pattern.

2. Stream from deepest layer to superficial as a suspending, expanding ball of waves rippling up from the depths

3. Glide from deepest layers through to the surface with rotating, spiraling movements.

UNWINDING PATTERNS

1. Focus on an inertial patterned area. Let your body begin to unwind the tissue around it internally.

2. Follow the unwinding as a witness without engaging in the movement.

3. Follow the unwinding until it comes to stillness.

MIDLINE AND STILLNESS

1. Focus on your midline. Let the stillness of this fulcrum deepen and recalibrate your matrix.

2. Witness whatever internal movement happens without engaging and moving with it.

3. Deepen into your stillness.

RECALIBRATION AND RENEWAL

As we go through our day and move repetitively, pushing and pulling against gravity, we align our microfibril/organized water matrix to the fulcrum of our movements. This alignment begins to hold us against gravity and reduce the matrix's complex mutability. By doing the Basic Sequence (pg. 213), we reopen that complexity and return our fascial matrix to its mutable, mobile state. In order to recalibrate and renew the diversity of the microfibril/organized water matrix, we must bring our reference point back to our midline. So, after performing the Basic Sequence and exploring other aspects of our fascial matrix, we should always return to the midline, our fulcrum of stillness.

GLIDING TO MIDLINE

1. Lying on your back with your legs and arms extended, focus on gliding your internal matrix from your extremities to your midline. Glide from the fingertips of one arm to your midline. Pause in the stillness of your midline. Glide from the fingertips of your other arm to your midline. Pause again in the stillness of your midline.

2. Glide from the toes of one leg to your midline. Pause in the stillness of your midline. Glide from the toes of your other leg to your midline, then pause, once again, in the stillness of your midline

3. Glide from the edges of your torso to your midline. Pause in the stillness of your midline. Glide from your head to your midline. Pause in the stillness of your midline.

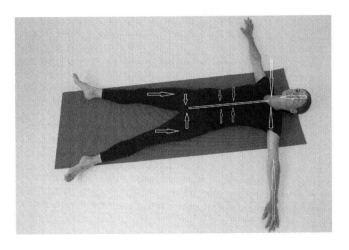

Gliding to midline

STREAMING FROM MIDLINE

1. From your midline, follow the streaming out from your midline and let it spiral through your microfibril/organized water matrix wherever it goes. Allow your streaming to move your body in slow, spiral motions.

2. Hold your awareness at the midline as your streaming recalibrates your matrix, until your body moves back into stillness. Allow yourself to deepen into the stillness of your renewed system.

CHAPTER 23
FASCIAL CONDUCTION

HANDS-ON PRACTICE

INTRODUCTION

Now that we have learned about the structure and field of our fascial system, moved and explored our internal matrix, and connected our body through its fractal relationships, let's turn our attention to working the bioelectric field with our hands.

This hands-on practice is called *Fascial Conduction*. Whether or not you are a professional hands-on practitioner, you can use these techniques to enhance the capacity of the matrix. If you have experience as a massage therapist, physical therapist, bodywork practitioner or energy worker, your own expertise and techniques will be enhanced by the practice of Fascial Conduction. If you are interested in becoming a Fascial Conduction practitioner, then you will want to participate in workshops on Fascial Conduction, as well as work with other practitioners to broaden and deepen your skills as a practitioner.

Fascial Conduction works at the structural and field levels, using the structure of the matrix of both client and practitioner to enhance the conductive capacity of the fascial layers. By working at certain levels of tissue, Fascial Conduction can use the fractal relationships to move through the macro-structure to the micro-structure, and through the levels of field, to the quantum level. By creating more complexity in the microfibril/organized water matrix and opening up inertial patterns in the body, a hands-on practitioner can enhance the adaptation, vitality and potency of the client's body. By dancing with the fascial matrix, we can enliven and integrate the body's coherent resonator of consciousness.

Fascial Conduction is a system that contacts the impulses and patterns that flow through the microfibril/organized water matrix, following their ripples and gliding them into all the tissue layers of the body. It contacts both the physical and energetic impulses that are conducted through the bioelectric matrix, creating a coherent connection felt as a current through the practitioner's hands.

In the work of Fascial Conduction, instead of focusing on specific tissues, techniques and patterns, we put our attention to the relationship between the tissue, rhythms and patterns. By focusing on the qualities of the matrix and arrangement of the microfibrils, practitioners can be the witness to the interactions of systems, polarities, movements and rhythms. As these qualities and arrangements become more dynamic and mutable, we enhance the information network of the whole body and create greater internal and external conscious awareness.

Fascial Conduction provides guidelines for how to contact and move the internal matrix as well as letting the practitioner use their own expertise and techniques to enliven the matrix. Whether direct or indirect, all outside techniques of working with fascia can be used as they relate to the qualities and wave patterns of the matrix. By concentrating on the quality of the tissue, using the sensations of viscosity, pulsation and glide, the practitioner is able to connect with the rhythms of the client and feel places of inertia and congestion. The practitioner will use the parts of the matrix that are open and moving to inform the places that are not.

By touching and mirroring the qualities of density, fluidity, glide, compartmentalization, conductivity, suspension and coherence, we can increase the diversity of choices in the matrix. By opening up habitual inertial patterns, Fascial Conduction is able to bring the body back to a being vital, potent, whole organism.

The work of Fascial Conduction draws on the contact and movement of the fascia to awaken the parasympathetic component of the nervous system. As the practitioner caresses the internal matrix, mirroring its fluid and wave patterns, this allows the whole organism of the client to deeply relax and recalibrate.

The work of Fascial Conduction is constantly being informed by the client as well as by the practitioner. The work is conducive to many types of cranial and fascial modalities, as it does not follow a specific technique sequence. It is a field of intention that draws on the practitioner's natural and learned talents to feel deeply into the voice of the fascial matrix.

MAKING CONTACT: MATRIX TO MATRIX

As we begin to contact the fascial matrix of our client, we must first align ourselves with our own bioelectric matrix, so that we can connect matrix to matrix.

Because we have our own patterns that are mirrors of our traumas, injuries and habits of movement, we want to neutralize our personal story in order to work with our clients. We use our midline to do this. So, before touching our client's matrix, we find our midline and let our tissues settle into this place of neutral.

Once we have found our midline, and settled into it, we can begin to feel the ebb and flow of our liquid crystalline matrix moving the around our midline. As this flow pulses through our microfibril/organized water pathways, we draw our concentration to the matrix pathways in our hands. We can feel the bioelectric field in our hands as a subtle rhythmic pulsation, spreading and opening from the palms out to the fingertips.

This opening of sensation in the hands feels like a spreading and suspension, moving out of the coherence in the palms. Letting out fingers extend away from each other, we can feel the suspension through the wrist and forearm, up to the shoulders. Now we are in our bioelectric matrix and can make contact with our client.

Most of the time, we make contact with our client through clothing or a covering between us. This helps to limit the sensory stimulus that pressure excites on the skin. By bypassing the sensory nervous system, we contact the dynamic matrix without the central nervous system interfering with commentary about the pressure and warmth of sensation.

We make contact with the full hand or fingertips, usually with multiple points of contact. This engages the three-dimensional matrix and contacts compressive and tensile forces. Once we are engaged with the client's bioelectric matrix, we may begin to use one, two or multi-point holds to glide or stream impulses into their tissue.

EXPLORATION 65: FINDING THE MICROFIBRIL/ORGANIZED WATER MATRIX IN OUR HANDS

Find a comfortable sitting position and settle into your body. Bring your focus to your internal matrix. Feel the vibration and relationship within the matrix. Feel the microfibrils and organized water that make up the matrix. Feel the vibrational pulses through the matrix pathways.

Follow the sensation of the matrix to the midline. Feel the stillness in the midline. Move your focus out from the midline through the matrix pathways, following them through the shoulders down the arms to the hands.

Feel the matrix in your hands. Feel the fibril/organized water matrix out to the fingertips. Place your fingertips together. Notice the connection in the matrix between your left and right hand. Notice the information being exchanged between your fingertips. Now release your fingertips.

Now you are ready to contact your client's matrix.

CONTACTING THE STRUCTURE

In Fascial Conduction, we are connecting with the liquid crystalline matrix that shapes and forms our client's body, conducts their signature rhythms and adapts to the inputs of their internal and external environments. We can contact a specific layer of the matrix, a specific quality of the matrix, or the crystalline memory in the matrix.

Once we have made contact with intention, we use direct and/or indirect methods to begin to move, liquefy, complexify and balance our client's matrix back to its alignment with the midline fulcrum, enhancing its mutability. As we dance with one area of the matrix, it guides us to the direction of movement that will open and reconnect inertial patterns back into the whole matrix. As we open and rebalance one part of our client's matrix, we can feel the pull of other areas in their matrix that are a part of the whole body's imbalance.

We work with the different fractal layers of the matrix, from the shape and form of the matrix in the superficial sleeve, to the suspension of the matrix surrounding the organs, to the rhythmic pulsations moving through the organized water within and between the microfibrils, to the conductive capacity of the system. By shifting the habitual patterns of our client's matrix, we reconnect their communication matrix network, enhancing the vitality and potency of the whole system.

There are many ways to contact the structural layers in the matrix. In Fascial Conduction there are three movement patterns we use to enhance the mutability, mobility and adaptability of the matrix. They include (1) the slide and glide, (2) the lemniscate or figure eight, and (2) the compress and glide.

- **Slide and glide**—moving the fascial matrix between the other tissues in the body in any direction, engaging the three-dimensional structure

- **Figure eight**—moving in and out of a center fulcrum in a three-dimensional figure eight.

- **Compress and glide**—compressing with one hand while gliding down the tensile forces until you come to a place of compression, then holding that compressive force while gliding down another direction of tensile force.

WAYS TO CONTACT THE STRUCTURE

- Use 30° angle to pull up the slack
- Glide the tissues slowing and evenly
- Move into deeper layers
- Follow longitudinal, horizontal, rotational
- and spiral movements
- Find compressive and tensile factors
- Witness and follow the fascial movement
- Move fascial layers in multiple directions
- Engage client in active awareness and
- movement

EFFECTS OF CONTACTING THE STRUCTURE

- Create greater space and mobility
- Complexify the microfibril/organized water matrix
- Enhance the adaptability of the tissue
- Release inertial patterns
- Restore vitality and potency
- Reconnect the matrix to the whole organism
- Restore the dynamic of tensile and compressive forces

CONTACTING THE FIELD

When we contact the matrix field, we are contacting the resonant field held in the microfibril/organized water matrix. Our attention is drawn to the vibrational, rhythmic signature wave patterns of our clients. When in the field we draw upon the mesodermic field of mutability and stem cell memory to open the conductive field in the matrix, increase the flow of information within the tissues, and enliven our client's resonant capacity. We can work at the surface, drawing the wave pattern through the deeper layers, or we can direct our intention to specific vibrational rhythms such as the breath, heartbeat, cranial rhythm, or longer, slower rhythms.

Once we have contacted the field and feel the undulations of the organism, we use direct and indirect methods of holding, streaming, following and returning to enhance the flow of information and coherence in the organism. When we feel the shifting of the field through heat, unwinding or changes in the vibrational pattern, we hold to let the system recalibrate and open its field of relationship. Once an area has settled and finished its work, we shift our focus to another inertial pattern. Once we have worked the areas of concern, we complete the work by sending an impulse through our client's matrix to reconnect all of the information pathways.

We work with the internal vibrational patterns, as well as with their relationship to both the practitioner's patterns and the electromagnetic patterns of the surrounding environment. As the client's vibrational pattern becomes strong, resilient and integrated throughout the microfibril/organized water matrix, the client's ability to choose what external vibrational patterns they want to engage is increased. The client's signature wave pattern becomes attuned to the external environment, exchanging information with the outside without being disturbed by the external environmental field.

WAYS TO CONTACT THE FIELD

- Use two-hand contact
- Settle lightly into tissues
- Be the witness
- Contact vibrational pulsations within the microfibril/organized water matrix
- Feel pull of the bioelectric matrix
- Feel suspension, floating and wave patterns
- Find the potency and reserves that reside in the field
- Let the client's tissue rise into your touch and move you through its patterns

EFFECTS OF CONTACTING THE FIELD

- Restore balanced reciprocal tension
- Enliven the matrix
- Restore complexity of conductive pathways
- Enhance potency
- Increase adaptability
- Increase the flow of information

CREATING AN IMPULSE

When we have made contact with our client's fascial structure or field, we introduce a small impulse of pressure or pull to engage their matrix. This impulse can be as subtle as our intention with physical pressure, or as specific as a hooking into their matrix and pulling it very gently in a certain direction. We can use an impulse throughout a session to find inertial patterns or assess the mutability and changes in our client's matrix.

In the structure this impulse initiates the shifting of tensile and compressive forces, starting the dance of rebalancing, creating suspension and support in our client. As we direct or follow these forces and movements within our client's matrix through streaming, our impulses continue to inform and shift the connections and mobility of their matrix.

When we work in the field, our impulse is a drop in the still waters, initiating a wave pattern through our client's matrix. This impulse streams with the signature wave pattern of our client. These ripples in the wave pattern excite ionic forces, helping them to rebalance coherence and suspension in the fractal system.

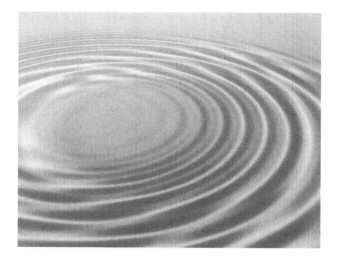

Creating an impulse

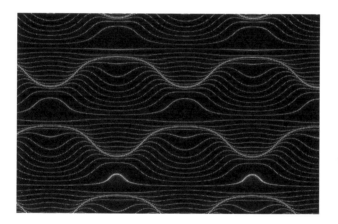

Impulse on wave patterns

STREAMING

Once we have engaged the matrix of our client with our impulse, we can follow or direct this impulse through streaming. *Streaming* is following or directing the impulse through the microfibril/organized water matrix as it shifts and changes in response to the impulse, changing the tensile or compressive forces and wave patterns in the organism.

When working with the structure, streaming can be multidirectional, shifting direction as the changes follow the impulse within the matrix. If we are working with slide and glide, we will take hold at one part of the matrix with our lower hand, gently pulling away from that hold and streaming until we feel a significant tug from the lower hand. Then we hold with the upper hand and stream the opposite way by moving the matrix with the lower hand. As we slide and glide in this way we open the matrix to complexify and increase its mobility. We slide and glide in a vertical, horizontal, diagonal or spiral directions, we engage different layers and levels of our client's bioelectric matrix.

When working with the figure eight technique, we open our client's matrix at a micro-movement level, finding a center fulcrum from which to circle around in multiple directions. The figure eight streams in all directions within the sphere of the fulcrum, opening and enhancing the buoyancy and suspension around the fulcrum.

When we are working with the compressive and tensile forces, we give a slight compression to one area, then stream and glide from that place until we meet another compressive junction. We let go of the first compression, hold the compressive junction we have found, and stream away from it. We continue this shifting of compression and streaming down the tensile forces, opening and enhancing the adaptability of the matrix.

When we are working at the field level, we let the impulse move a wave pattern through the matrix, and we follow this streaming of the wave pattern through our client's body. As we listen and follow the wave patterns of their integrated matrix, we begin to reengage their inertial patterns back into their signature wave pattern.

FASCIAL CONDUCTION PRACTICE

WHAT TO EXPECT AS A CLIENT

If you are receiving a fascial conduction session you will be asked about your health history and the concerns that you have at the time of the session. You will lie down on a comfortable massage table with your clothes on. It is useful to where loose fitting clothing and no jewelry. The practitioner will usually begin at your feet giving a gentle impulse at your ankles up the body. Once the conductive pattern is assessed, the practitioner will work on different areas of the body usually with a two point contact, using hands or fingers or forearm. This contact can be on the front and back of the body, side by side or in diagonals on the body. The touch is light and engaging. The practitioner's hands will move with the movement of your matrix, not along the contours of the body. You will begin to relax as your body settles into the conversation between your matrix and the practitioner's matrix. A deep sense of relaxation will usually occur as well as different sensations that will come and go as your inertial patterns are reintegrated into your matrix. The effect may include a shift in discomfort, pain and stiffness, a sense of openness, buoyancy and suspension, and a sense of integration and wholeness.

WHAT FOLLOWS ARE SOME BASIC APPROACHES TO HANDS-ON FASCIAL CONDUCTION PRACTICE FOR THE PRACTITIONER.

As the practitioner, it is important to find your midline and matrix before putting your hands on your client. Once you have settled into your own matrix system, you can assess your client's matrix by putting a gently impulse into their matrix at the ankles. As you follow the conductive pathways up the body to the head, you will notice places of slowness, areas blocking the flow of the impulse, deviation from the vertical impulse, conductive pulls into certain areas or differences in the quality of conductive flow in the layers of the matrix. Once you have assessed the matrix, begin at the area where you have found some differences and use the skills described below to reintegrate inertial patterns, balance quality differences and enliven the areas of congestion. When you have finished reassess the conductivity in the matrix through another impulse at the ankles.

CONTACTING MATRIX TO MATRIX

Bring your awareness to your midline, following it from the top of your head, through the front of your sphenoid, front of your spine, front of your sacrum, and to your coccyx. Maintain your awareness of your midline while moving through your internal matrix to your hands. Feel the bioelectric channels in your hands as they reach out to the surface of your palms. Gently place your hands on your client, feeling when your matrix connects with theirs. You may feel a subtle pull into the surface you are touching or just a sense of connection, tissue to tissue.

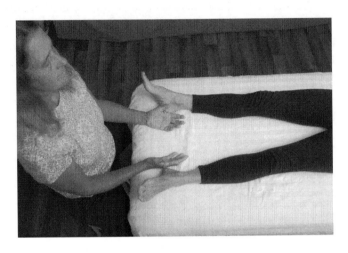

Sensing the matrix in your palms

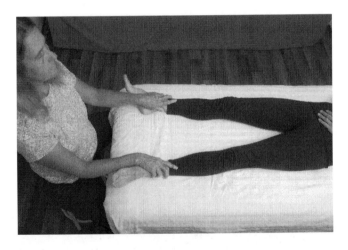

Contacting your client's matrix

SLIDE AND GLIDE (IMPULSE AND STREAM)

At knee: Place your hands on either side of the knee, hold the matrix with one hand (distal side), gently pull away with other hand (proximal side) until the matrix engages (this creates the impulse). Glide matrix with both hands in the direction of the hand that is pulling away (proximally) until you feel resistance in the other hand (this creates the streaming). Now hold the matrix with hand pulling away (proximal side) while gently pulling away with other hand (distal side). When the matrix engages, glide the matrix gently with both hands back down (distally) until you feel resistance. Go back and forth, feeling the increase of mobility in the matrix layers in the joint capsule. Try to bring in other layers of the matrix that surround the ligaments, joint capsule and musculature.

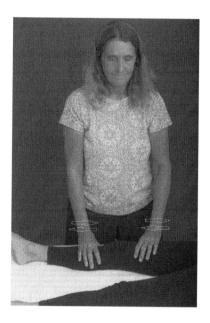

Slide and Glide at knee

At hip: Place your hands on the outside (lateral) and inside (medial) of the hip bone on the front side of your client's body (illium). Hold the matrix on the outside of the hip while gently pulling around the edge of the hip bone with the inside hand, until the matrix engages. Glide around the hip bone from outside to inside with both hands until you feel resistance. Then hold the inside hand while gently pulling around the edge hip bone to the outside, until the matrix engages. Then glide the matrix around the hip bone from inside to outside until you feel resistance, going back and forth and increasing the length of the glide. Try to engage the deeper layers of tissue around the ilium.

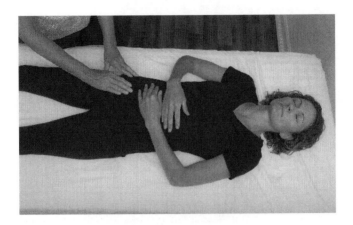

Gliding around the illium

At shoulder: Place your hands on the front (anterior) and back (posterior) of the shoulder (on either side of the head of the humerus). Gently pull your hands away from each other until the matrix engages. Glide in circular and spiral motions around the shoulder. Feel the opening of the multidirectional matrix around the shoulder.

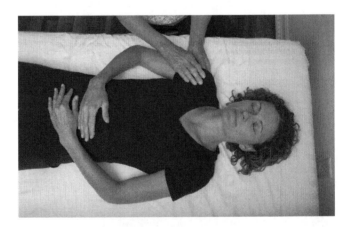

Gliding the shoulder

Slide and glide in the field: At any of the previous areas, start with same hand contact, feeling the contact with the bioelectric matrix field. Feel the pull between your hands, witnessing and following the streaming of movement in the matrix as it recalibrates and moves wave motion through it, increasing its motility.

REESTABLISHING THE MIDLINE FULCRUM

FIGURE EIGHT, LEMNISCATE

At the spine: Place your hands on the front and back of the client's body at the midline, your front hand at the sternum, you back hand over the spine. Gently press your hands towards each other until the matrix engages (impulse). Move the matrix (streaming) in a figure eight out from the midline, first out to one side of the vertebra and sternum, until you feel resistance, then circle around and back to the midline. Move the matrix between your hands to the other side until you feel resistance, then circle around and back to the midline. Move out diagonally from the sternum until you feel resistance, then circle back to the midline. Move out the other side in the opposite diagonal until you feel resistance, then circle back to the midline, maintaining the figure eight. Let the diagonal move out in different angles from the midline. Repeat this as you shift your hand placement to be at the diaphragm and vertebra, abdomen and vertebra, and lower abdomen and sacrum.

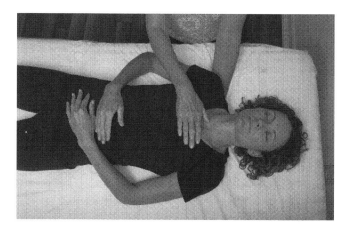

Figure 8 around midline

At the hips: Place your hands on the outside (lateral) of the client's hips, contacting the ilium. Gently press your hands toward each other until the matrix engages (impulse). Move the matrix (streaming) in a figure eight pattern with both hands from one hip to the other. Let the midline of the pelvic region be the midpoint fulcrum of the figure eight. Let the figure eight move in multi directions, keeping the same midline fulcrum point. Try to engage deeper layers of the matrix by deepening the level of your contact.

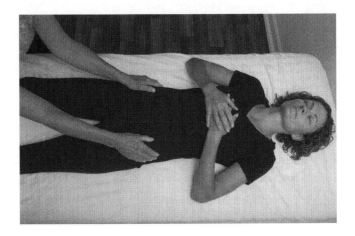

Figure 8 through hips

Figure eight in the field: Starting with either of the contacts above, engage the matrix and witness the pulsation within it from the midline out and back. Feel the wave motion build and move out of the midline. Once full, move back to the center point of the midline. Follow and witness the ebb and flow of the wave motion in and out of the midline.

BALANCING RECIPROCAL TENSIONS

MOVING COMPRESSIVE AND TENSILE FORCES

At the ribcage: Place your hands on the upper and lower ribs on one side of your client. Create a slight compression with your lower hand until the matrix engages (impulse). Glide (streaming) with your upper hand in whatever way the matrix wants to glide. When your upper hand meets resistance (compression), release the compression from the lower hand, hold the compression with your upper hand, and glide with the lower hand in the direction of easiest movement until you come to another compressive force. Continue to move from the compressive force, gliding (streaming) down the tensile forces, to the next compressive force. Shift the positions of your hands to other parts of the ribs so you can enliven the biotensegrity of the area.

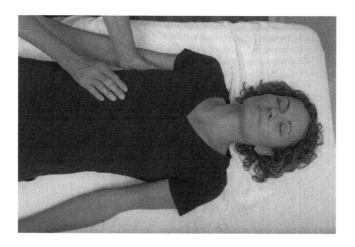

Gliding tensile and compressive forces

At the forearm: Place your hands across the back (posterior side) of your client's forearm, above the wrist and below the elbow. Create a slight pull or compression with one hand until the matrix engages (impulse), and glide (streaming) in rotational directions through the tensile forces with the other hand until you feel resistance. Hold this resistance and glide the tensile forces with rotation and spirals with the other hand. Engage deeper layers with greater rotation, feeling the area between the forearm bones (ulna and radius). Shift hand positions to engage more of the compressive and tensile forces.

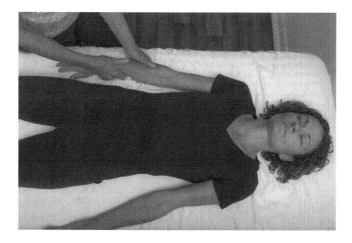

Rotational gliding into deeper layers

249

In the field: Placing hands on either side of a joint or specific area, feel the coherent forces pulling your hands together. Witness the coherence. Find the forces of suspension that pull your hands away from each other, following that pull away to the point where is disengages. Release back to where you feel the suspending forces and witness the opening and shifting wave patterns in the matrix.

APPLYING MASSAGE TECHNIQUES TO FASCIAL CONDUCTION

DIRECT AND INDIRECT METHODS

There are many hands-on massage and bodywork techniques that address the fascia and affect its structure and field within the body. Many of these massage techniques are taught in basic massage certification programs. By going through a certification you will gain a greater sensitivity and understanding of the tissue layers and what techniques apply to what systems. Once your hands are experienced in feeling the different tissue systems, and once you know how to apply different techniques to them, you can differentiate between direct and indirect methods. You can begin to distinguish between working the structure and working the field.

The direct methods in massage and bodywork are techniques that work directly on the soft tissue, manipulating and shifting its length, viscosity, buoyancy and multidimensionality. By taking the tissue and moving it in varying directions, these techniques can inform the fascia and shift its balanced reciprocal tension. These methods use force, friction and pull to directly change the shape and form of fascial tissue.

The indirect methods used in massage and bodywork are the techniques that contact tissue layers and follow the movement and unwinding patterns in the tissue. The indirect methods use contact to invite tissue to move and change. These methods include holding, vibrating and conducting tissue without direct manipulation.

DIRECT MODALITIES THAT CONTACT THE STRUCTURE

- Deep tissue massage
- Connective tissue massage
- Structural integration
- Myofascial release
- Neuromuscular therapy
- Trigger point therapy
- Rolfing

INDIRECT MODALITIES THAT CONTACT THE STRUCTURE

- Cranial sacral therapy
- Somato-emotional release
- Fascial unwinding
- Zero balancing

MODALITIES THAT CONTACT THE FIELD

- Biodynamic cranial therapy
- Polarity therapy
- Energetic meridian therapies
- Acupressure
- Chakra work
- Energy work
- Continuum

THINGS TO REMEMBER IN HANDS-ON PRACTICE

- The stronger the impulse the weaker the response
- Be specific and know exactly where you are working on the body, including anatomy and level of depth
- Move the tissue slowly, both in the pressure changes and movement through the internal spaces
- Listen to the tissue and let your own matrix determine the pressure and direction of your touch
- Notice how the matrix is moving in areas you are not touching
- Use multiple contact points to engage more of the matrix
- Assess the mobility and motility of the matrix before and after your hands-on session

---

HANDS-ON PRACTICE ADDRESSING MATRIX QUALITIES: TECHNIQUES FOR WORKING STRUCTURE/FIELD

When working the matrix we create intention around the quality we want to enliven and enhance using specific skills to address them. We begin by engaging the matrix using an impulse at the feet and streaming the impulse up the body. We listen to where we feel that quality is inhibiting the integration of the matrix, and go to that area to begin. We also use information from talking with the client, and a structural assessment to inform our intention. As we begin to impulse and stream in an area, using the movement patterns of slide and glide, figure eight, and compressive and tensile forces, along with other appropriate massage techniques, we notice the quality changes and the dissolving of inertial patterns, integrating areas back into the whole organism.

QUALITY OF DENSITY, GEL/SOL

Begin by finding your midline, then your matrix in your palms (see pg. 243), and place your hands above your client's ankles. Gently compress with your hands until you engage the matrix (impulse). Stream your impulse up the client's body with a slight movement upward, and notice where the impulse stops, slows down or deviates from the midline. Use your assessment skills to notice the areas where there is more resistance and less ability to penetrate, limited range of motion, or no movement at all. Determine what is the densest area and begin to work in that area.

AT DENSER AREAS

Begin by putting hands around the denser area and compress slightly until the matrix engages (impulse).

Notice the degree of density and lack of movement in the area.

Start with a longitudinal slide and glide (see pg. 244, streaming) at the superficial matrix layer.

Begin to deepen your slide and glide into the next level of fascia. Shift to a diagonal and horizontal slide and glide in the area.

Find the fulcrum (center) of the density and use figure eight micro-movements (see pg. 247) directly into it.

Keep your contact with the matrix and witness the unwinding and enlivening in the tissue. Notice the change in the degree of density.

Work with the tensile and compressive forces (see pg. 248) around the dense area.

Shift your attention to the field and feel the wave patterns as they spiral and ripple through the dense area.

Hold and witness the enlivenment of the liquid crystalline matrix as it reintegrates the dense area into the whole matrix.

Use your own massage techniques to shift from the gel of density to the sol of fluidity.

Slide and glide (see pg. 244) the area back into the whole matrix.

Move to other compressed, dense areas.

Finish the session with slide and glide at the superficial fascia.

QUALITY OF GLIDE

Begin by finding your midline, then your matrix in your palms (see pg. 244), and place your hands above your client's ankles. Gently compress with your hands until you engage the matrix (impulse). Stream your impulse up the body with a slight movement upward, and notice where the impulse stops, slows down or deviates from the midline. Use your assessment skills to notice areas where there is little or no movement, or where the movement is sticky or choppy, and being to work in that area of limited slide and glide.

AREAS WITH LIMITED SLIDE AND GLIDE

Begin by making contact with two hands on either side of area with little or no internal movement.

Slide and glide (see pg. 244) from your impulse hand to the other and back, gliding longitudinally through the area.

Deepen contact to slide and glide the deeper layers of the matrix. Slide and glide horizontally and diagonally.

Slide and glide superficial layer over bones. Slide and glide deeper layers under bones.

Follow the slide and glide in spiral and multidirectional patterns. Let the matrix determine where you use the slide and glide movements.

Stay connected with your client's matrix and witness the matrix gliding.

Change the placement of your hands, engage the matrix (impulse), and slide and glide (streaming) in new positions on the body, noticing other impaired areas and the slide and glide up the body.

Flex and extend the client's foot while gliding with your upper hand at their hip to integrate glide in lower extremities.

Gently extend the client's arm away from their torso while gliding at upper torso to increase glide in multiple layers of shoulder.

Use your own massage techniques that enhance glide.

Create another impulse at the feet to feel the increase in slide and glide.

Slide and glide wherever there is still resistance.

Finish with slide and glide in the client's superficial matrix.

QUALITY OF LAYERING

Begin by finding your midline, then your matrix in your palms (see pg. 243), and place your hands above your client's ankles. Gently compress with your hands until you engage the matrix (impulse). Stream your impulse up the body with a slight movement upward, and notice where the impulse stops, slows down or deviates from the midline. Use your assessment skills to notice which layer of the matrix glides the most and which glides the least. If the matrix glides easily in the back of the body (posteriorly), work the front (anterior) side. If it glides easily on the outside (laterally), work the inside (medially).

LAYERS THAT HAVE LIMITED GLIDE

Begin where there is less movement or glide.

Slide and glide (see pg. 244) longitudinally to increase the glide in that part of the matrix.

Slide and glide horizontally and in rotation, working above and below the bones to reach layers of the matrix.

Use micro-movements of slide and glide (*very* tiny slide and glide) in areas that are sticky and resistant.

Find specific layers of fascia around muscles, between muscles, around bones or around organs, then slide and glide through the planes in which they are found.

Work compressive and tensile forces (see pg. 248) through each layer to rebalance reciprocal tension.

Take the client's matrix between your hands and pull it gently away from the area of stickiness, suspending and opening between the layers.

Follow and witness the unwinding and reintegrating of the matrix's layers.

Use other appropriate massage techniques to individuate tissue layers.

Slide and Glide the area to reintegrate the layers to the whole matrix.

BALANCING RECIPROCAL TENSION OF COMPRESSIVE/TENSILE FORCES,

COHERENCE/SUSPENSION

Begin by finding your midline, then your matrix in your palms (see pg. 243), and place your hands above your client's ankles. Gently compress with your hands until you engage the matrix (impulse). Stream your impulse up the body with a slight movement upward, and notice where the impulse stops, slows down or deviates from the midline. Use your assessment skills to notice where the matrix is compressed and contained, or where the matrix is stretched out too far. Notice where the matrix is not responding to the shift in pressure and tensile forces but holding its push or pull. Notice where the streaming goes around areas or doesn't engage with the integrated matrix.

AREAS OF COMPRESSION, OVERSTRETCH OR IMMOBILITY

Begin at an area of compression, overstretch or immobility.

Compress slightly on the chosen area to engage the matrix and move down the tensile forces until you feel the next compression (see pg. 248). Let go of the first compression and glide down the second compressed place you came to.

Continue to compress and glide down the tensile forces.

Notice areas which are over-compressed and that don't respond to the streaming. Create suspension in the area and feel the layers of the matrix rebalance.

Glide toward the compressed area until you feel coherence. Then glide away, feeling the coherence holding.

Notice areas that are stretched taut and thinned out. Create coherence by gently engaging the matrix on either side of the area and pulling the matrix toward the center of the area.

Use slide and glide (see pg. 244) in the area to balance the coherence and suspension.

Use other appropriate massage techniques to balance the reciprocal tensions.

Slide and glide the larger superficial matrix to integrate back into the whole.

INERTIAL PATTERNS

Begin by finding your midline, then your matrix in your palms (see pg. 243), and place your hands above your client's ankles. Gently compress with your hands until you engage the matrix (impulse). Stream your impulse up the body with a slight movement upward, and notice where the impulse stops, slows down or deviates from the midline. Use your assessment skills to notice areas of density, lack of tissue definition, limited range of motion, or where injury or trauma have occurred.

INERTIAL PATTERNED AREAS

Begin at an area of injury, lack of movement or sensation, or an area of pain and discomfort.

Slide and glide (see pg. 244) outside area of the inertial pattern, gliding up to the area and back. Increase the glide into the inertial area.

Find the center fulcrum in the inertial area and begin with figure eights (see pg. 247) in micro-movements from center of the fulcrum in all directions.

Widen your figure eight to encompass both inertial and open areas.

Find the over-compressed area in the inertial pattern and move the tensile forces away from it, until you feel resistance.

Slide and glide in the inertial area to assess if the inertial pattern has reintegrated into the whole matrix.

Repeat these methods through the layers in the area to clear and rebalance the full matrix.

Use appropriate massage techniques that can stimulate the tissue systems in the area to integrate them into the whole matrix.

Finish by slide and glide in the client's larger superficial matrix to reintegrate into the whole.

EFFECTS OF QUALITY INTENTION IN HANDS-ON PRACTICE

- Increase sponginess and resilience in the matrix
- Increase mobility and motility within the matrix
- Increase complexity of the microfibril/organized water matrix
- Create an integrated interconnected matrix
- Enhance the ability to resonate wave patterns to every cell
- Increase coherence and suspension in the matrix
- Enhance bioelectric capacity in the organized water
- Enhance conductive capacity
- Enhance healing capacity
- Enhance potency and vitality
- Reduce restrictions from over-compression or repetitive patterns of conduction
- Increase adaptability in the whole organism

LEVELS OF CONDUCTIVITY

When we address some of the qualities of our client's matrix, enhancing its healthy dynamic nature, we increase its bioelectric capacity. This includes giving more pathways for wave patterns to move, more stability within the ever-changing matrix, more ability to inform the cells of the organism's activities, and more integration within the whole organism. When these aspects are enhanced our client's matrix is better able to differentiate between its internal conduction and the external electromagnetic and bioelectric forces. A strong conductive medium is more capable of protecting and deflecting incoming conductive forces. A strong conductive medium is more capable of protecting itself from other conductive influences and can override those forces, reducing their negative influence on the integrated system.

By enhancing the conductive capacity of our client's matrix, we give her a stronger, integrated wholeness that supports their heath, vitality and potency. By enhancing the levels of conductivity, we create a protective barrier between the internal and external environments. This allows our client's body to choose what external wave patterns will pulsate through its pathways, and what external wave patterns it will shed off its surface. When our client choose to engage, the strong conductive pathways take in the wave patterns, informing every cell of this stimulus. When they choose not to engage, our surface matrix can shed the wave patterns surrounding us, creating safety and protection for all the cells.

ABILITY TO RESONATE SIGNATURE WAVE TO EXTERNAL MATRIX

When our levels of conduction are strengthened, our ability to resonate and engage with the external world increases. We are able to notice and sense many of the conductive patterns in our environment (including the electromagnetic field of Earth, bioelectric fields of all living things, artificial electric fields from cell towers, electricity grids, and electrical and quantum fields from the sun, planets and other fields that reach the Earth). We can then choose how to engage or disengage with these fields. With this strong conductive base, we are able to resonate our own signature wave into the environment, influencing its wave pattern relationships.

With this heightened conductive relationship, we are able to interconnect with different patterns of resonance that come from all living things, the Earth, and the universe. As we choose to resonate with other external fields, we begin to experience the integrated wholeness of the universe. As we shift from the limited access of our internal matrix to access the universal vibrations, we extend out of our survival neurological mechanisms of separation and become integrated with the bigger vibratory organism of the vast universe.

CHAPTER 24
CASE STUDIES

To understand the techniques and effects Fascial Conduction, I have included four case studies to provide more detailed information about working with specific symptoms and health issues. I have chosen four very different clients with unique concerns, and I have shown how doing the hands-on work of Fascial Conduction, along with self-practice exercises for the client, affects both the specific symptoms and overall health and well-being of the client.

CASE STUDY 1—EXCESS FLUID, TIGHTENING THE BOUNDARIES

It is important to understand that more energy is not necessarily better. When we have an overflowing of energy and enthusiasm that expands our boundaries past where our bodies can contain them, an imbalance can develop between inward and outward experiences, between rest and activity, and between expression and reflection. Here is an example of how the work found in *Moving Matrix* can help to balance the reciprocal tension of the matrix, bringing in strong boundaries that create protection and safety.

Sasha came to her first session with me overflowing with energy and enthusiasm. She had problems staying centered and calm. She was continually moving and expressing herself without pause, her mind overactive and lacking any inward reflection. She had minor pains and discomforts, sometimes in her right arm and shoulder, and limited movement in her left hip. She was a dancer and teacher, looking to find more balance in her life between "doing and being."

When putting an impulse at Sasha's feet, I found that the conduction through the microfibril/organized water matrix pulsated at the superficial layer, with fluid wave movement pulsating at the deeper layers. The fluid wave movement was excessive, pulsing out to the surface, but not returning back to the midline. The movement of her wave pattern undulated throughout her body, but with very little ebb and flow, coherence, or pause at the midline. The boundaries of her field were disconnected and gave no distinction between her field and her surroundings.

I began working with Sasha's wave motions, bringing them into relationship with the midline. From the legs I initiated wave patterns to stream back into the deeper spaces of bone and marrow, keeping slight pressure to continue the internalization of her fluid patterns. Once the legs had shifted their wave pattern to a balanced ebb and flow, and once the boundaries provided by her superficial fascia were intact, I moved to the hips and worked with her horizontal diaphragm and pelvic bowl. Her pelvic floor was boundaried on the external side but disconnected on the internal side. After sliding and gliding the internal side, getting more conduction in the whole pelvic bowl, I worked with the pelvic floor matrix and brought it back into relationship with the whole matrix.

Next, I continued up the torso, gliding and streaming the wave patterns towards the midline, holding at the midline while letting the torso matrix reorganize. I worked the diagonal between the right shoulder and left leg to enliven the contralateral movement boundaries and to enhance coherence in the matrix. I worked with the left and right hemispheres of the brain to integrate to the midline, and I finished with holding the midline, letting the tissue continue to reorganize.

When impulsing at the end of the session through her feet, I found an amazingly intact matrix, strong boundaries and well established midline. As I continued to see Sasha we worked on some of her inertial patterns around organs, while her midline and boundaries have stayed interconnected with good coherence.

CASE STUDY 2—FULL-BODY DENSITY, CHANGING PERCEPTIONS

When we work with different bodies we perceive them through our own view of vitality and fluidity. What might feel like density for you might be a different view of fluidity for your client.

Bruce came in with some sore and tight areas of the right shoulder and left foot. When moving an impulse through him and feeling his matrix, I determined that his matrix was dense and tight with no mobility or motility. I saw his whole body as overly compressed with no suspension or glide.

I worked at increasing the sphere of movement in the matrix and gave specific time to the foot, where the plantar fascia was injured. I contacted the matrix in the foot and suspended the bones in the metatarsals. The Achilles and muscles attaching to it were also worked on, bringing suspension to the calcaneus bone, or heel bone.

For Bruce's shoulder, I worked with three of the rotator cuff attachments on the humerus, hoping to rebalance the matrix that supports them. I ended by moving the matrix from the head and suspending the neck.

The specific work seemed to increase glide in the area but had little effect on the glide and mobility of the whole matrix. His fascial matrix still seemed overly compresses with no suspension or space for movement or conduction. When I used an impulse to assess the shifts in the matrix, I found that changes in conductivity and glide were minimal. His matrix was still rigid and unresponsive.

We continued to work together monthly. The specific work seemed to make a difference in the small area of the matrix I was working with, but never seemed to change the amount of glide in the whole matrix. The fascial matrix was not complexifying or moving forward out of its original state. I began to reinterpret my assessments — from looking at the quantity of movement to looking at other qualities in his matrix. Although there was little internal movement in the matrix, the vitality and pulsation was shifting. In order to enhance vitality and conductivity, I needed to use micro-movements and streaming to connect to his microfibril/organized water matrix.

The different ways Bruce's internal matrix continued to evolve taught my hands a entirely different view of his matrix. I realized I had made assumptions about the amount of slack and internal movement to expect in his fascial matrix. My thinking was that the matrix had to have a certain amount of internal movement in order to complexify and conduct. But Bruce's limited internal movement was part of his makeup, and I could still enhance the matrix by working with micro-movements and streaming. This enhanced the qualities of vitality, conductivity and integration within the limited movement of his matrix. Thus I learned to suspend my own assumptions of how the matrix should feel and move, letting Bruce's matrix inform me of its nature while working with the qualities of his matrix that could shift.

CASE STUDY 3—EMBODIMENT, FINDING THE SIGNATURE WAVE

Our lives are driven, in many ways, by the complex workings of the central nervous system, so much so that our bodies can become servants to the needs of our mind's ruminations. We become desensitized to the experiences of the whole body and its matrix in order to use all of our available energy to understand complex questions. This, in turn, reduces the need for complexity in the microfibril/organized water matrix. With limited movement and activity we decrease our vitality, adaptability and whole body health. Finding balance between the neo cortex and the matrix is key.

Arlene came to see me to help her become more aware of her bodily sensations and how they influenced her perception. She is an academic and works overtime on grants, papers, lecturing and her books. She is a runner and meditator. She had some minor strains on her knees and her left hip from running, as well as some shoulder and arm discomfort from overuse of the computer.

I started by helping Arlene connect with her internal body. I did a guided meditation, helping her become aware of her microfibril/organized water matrix. From that somatic awareness she began to notice other sensations in her body. We used her imagination to begin to mark what body sensations connected with different memories, emotions or experiences. This gave her an internal source for her perceptions and turned her focus inside.

I then worked with her on the table. I began with an impulse at her feet and found that her matrix was very disorganized, so much so that the impulse moved chaotically through her system. Her midline was weak and the matrix had a pull toward her head, with very little flow back down the body. I began to slide and glide her matrix in the legs, opening and enlivening her joints and connecting the matrix from feet to hip. As the matrix began to enliven,

I could slide and glide deeper through the muscles, tendons, and into the periosteum of the bone. Her matrix began to conduct in multiple directions, connecting from superficial to deep, with a nice ebb and flow between layers.

I then worked at the hip, beginning at the external and internal sides of the hip bone, giving some support to the horizontal diaphragm and enlivening the pelvic matrix. I continued up the torso, suspending the matrix from the compressed posterior side to the disconnected anterior side. I worked in a figure eight motion to bring the torso matrix back into relationship with the midline, and I held the midline at the occiput.

I finished by holding the midline and letting the matrix reorganize. I asked Arlene to describe the difference in her internal sensation at that time. She was much more aware of the density and solidness of her body. She felt the midline and its relationship to the three dimensional internal space around it. She was amazed at her new sensations and was aware of her body's own internal dimensions.

I continued to work with Arlene, helping her to deepen her relationship with her internal matrix. She enjoyed doing some of the self-practice to further her internal sensing. She was particularly interested in feeling her signature wave and working at staying embodied during her busy academic schedule.

CASE STUDY 4: BILATERAL INJURY PROBLEMS, A COMPLEX SYSTEM

As we journey through our lives, our many experiences, mishaps and habits inform our matrix, as well as challenge it to adapt to the complexity of life. When working to reintegrate the matrix, this complexity in a client's cumulative life can be a maze of discovery that continues to recalibrate and adjust in compensational configurations into the present. It is important to suspend judgment and conclusions so that the unfolding of the recalibration can be followed.

When Carol came to see me, she had suffered a number of falls that had affected her left ankle so that the arch of her foot was painful whenever stepping down on it. She had been a dancer and teacher but was now unable to continue that part of her life. She had other compounding problems stemming from nerve damage caused by carbon monoxide poisoning.

Among other things, she desperately wanted to stabilize her ankle so she could return to her dance career.

When I put an impulse into her system, I felt disorganization in the three arches of her left foot, with conduction flow staying on the posterior side of her legs. Her right SI joint was fixed, along with a twisting of the flow through her solar plexus and right ribs. I felt how her whole body was configured around her disconnected left arch, so I began to work the left foot. I spent most of the time with a two-point hold, one anterior between the metatarsal bones and one at the bottom of the middle arch. By using micro-movements in the area I could feel the layers of the matrix unwind and shift, trying to recalibrate. I created suspension through the medial arch, then glided from the medial to lateral arch of the foot. I felt a push and pull in the matrix, reacting to my input. I continued to use smaller micro-movements until I made contact with the center of the issue. I glided from the connected matrix to the disconnected part until the push and pull subsided.

Next, I continued up the left leg, feeling compression on the posterior side, with containment on the lateral tendon of the hamstrings. I suspended the leg anteriorly to give more conduction through the center of the knee. I glided the matrix from the foot up the left leg, and I repeated on the right leg.

I worked on the hips, gliding the matrix through the SI joint, hip joint and medial/lateral iliac crest. I continued working up the body, finding disconnection at the solar plexus and right side of the ribs. Moving up to the head, I glided the dural tube and recalibrated the occiput to the sphenoid bone.

When I put in an impulse at the end of the session, I felt a new coherence in the conduction up the legs and integration in the flow through the hips. The right ribs and solar plexus stayed out of the conductive flow, and the inertial pattern in that area was informing new compensational patterns.

I continued to work with Carol for a number of weeks, working mostly with integrating the arches of her left foot, while spending a small amount of the time on the torso. The issues in the left foot continued to change location from the arches to the bottom of the calcaneus, to the instep of the foot below the large toe. As the foot recalibrated, the posterior containment in the left leg reduced and the hips began to rebalance.

The issues at the solar plexus and right ribs continued to inform the compensational patterns and held its fulcrum of disconnection. Because of the nerve damage on the right side from the carbon monoxide poisoning, the right side was an important place to enliven the matrix and give the area another way of integrating with the whole organism.

As I continue to work with the complex organization of Carol's system, I have suspend my conclusions about what the fulcrum of her problem is, and I try to work with whatever she brings to the session. Her ability to walk, stand and perform daily tasks has increased in both length of time and movement possibility, and her body's adaptable capacity has improved. Carol feels more stable in her legs and is beginning to look at practicing dance again. She reinjured her foot a number of times between sessions, but each time her ability to heal, recalibrate and integrate the matrix has quickened, and the old compensational patterns have not resurfaced. By working the matrix, and by enlivening its ability reengage itself back into the whole matrix, Carol's system is more equipped to meet the needs of her active life.

NOTES FOR FIGURES

CHAPTER 1

1. Shutterstock_230061868
2. Original drawing by Sue Sneddon
3. Shutterstock_208571902
4. Shutterstock_249531667
5. Original drawing by Sue Sneddon
6. Original drawing by Sue Sneddon
7. Wikimedia.com, https://flickr.com/photo/internetarchivebookimages/21285693065
8. Wikimedia.com, by Mypatob, File "Electromagnetic Wave"
9. Shutterstock_165798971
10. Shutterstock_304255052

CHAPTER 3

11. Original drawing by Sue Sneddon
12. Original drawing by Sue Sneddon
13. Shutterstock photo
14. Original drawing by Sue Sneddon
15. Original drawing by Sue Sneddon
16. Original drawing by Sue Sneddon

CHAPTER 4

17. Original drawing by Sue Sneddon

18. Original drawing by Sue Sneddon

19. Original drawing by Sue Sneddon

20. Original drawing by Sue Sneddon

21. Original drawing by Sue Sneddon

CHAPTER 5

22. Original drawing by Sue Sneddon

23. Original drawing by Sue Sneddon

24. Original drawing by Sue Sneddon

25. Original drawing by Sue Sneddon

26. Original drawing by Sue Sneddon

27. Shutterstock_164104628

28. Shutterstock_129464783

CHAPTER 6

29. Original drawing by Sue Sneddon

30. Shutterstock_199867760

CHAPTER 7

31. Original drawing by Sue Sneddon

32. Wikimedia.com, by Thomas Splettstoesser (www.scistyle.com)

33. Original drawing by Sue Sneddon

34. Original drawing by Sue Sneddon

CHAPTER 8

35. Original drawing by Sue Sneddon

36. Shutterstock_155676992

CHAPTER 9

37. Original drawings by Sue Sneddon
38. Original drawing by Sue Sneddon
39. Shutterstock_113758228
40. Original drawing by Sue Sneddon
41. Original drawing by Sue Sneddon

CHAPTER 10

42. Original drawing by Sue Sneddon
43. Original drawing by Sue Sneddon

CHAPTER 11

44. Photograph by author
45. Wikimedia: File: Broccoli DSCN4344.jpg.
46. Original drawings by Sue Sneddon
47. Original drawings by Sue Sneddon

CHAPTER 12

48. Shutterstock_175586489
49. Original drawing by Sue Sneddon
50. https://commons,wikimedia.org/w/index.php?curid=2336424
51. Original drawing by Sue Sneddon
52. Original drawing by Sue Sneddon
53. https://commons,wikimedia.org/w/index.php?curid=2030785

CHAPTER 13

54. Shutterstock_173060693

55. Wikimedia: File:Collagen-biosynthesis(en)png.

CHAPTER 16

56. http://cnx.org/content/co11496/1.6/, by Open Stax College, 419420421 Table 0401 updated.jpg.

CHAPTER 17

57. Original Drawing by Sue Sneddon

CHAPTER 18

58. Wikimedia.com, File: Conducting System en (CardioNetwork-sECGpedia).png

CHAPTER 22 & 23

All photos are originals by Cesar Carrasco.

IMPORTANT RESOURCES

Blechschmidt, E. *The Stages of Human Development before Birth,*Philadelphia: W.B. Saunders, l961.

Capra, Fritz, *The Hidden Connections,* New York: Doubleday, 2002.

Capra, Fritz, *The Web of Life,* New York: Anchor Books, 1996.

Conrad, Emily. *Life on Land, The story of Continuum,* Berkeley, Cal. North Atlantic Books, 2007.

Cohen, Bonnie Bainbridge, *Sensing, Feeling and Action,* Northampton, Mass: Contact Editions, 1993.

Gintis, Bonnie, *Engaging the Movement of Life ,*Berkeley, Ca. North Atlantic Books, 2007.

Grossinger, Richard, *Embryogenesis,* Berkeley, Ca., North Atlantic Books, 2000

Hitzmann, Sue, *The Melt Method,* Harper One, 2013.

Ho, Mae-Wan, *The Rainbow and the Worm, The Physics of Organisms,* World Scientific Publishing Company, New Jersey, 2008.

Ho, Mae-Wan *Living Rainbow H2O,* World Scientific Publishing Company, New Jersey, 2012

Hunt, Valerie, *Infinite Mind,* Malibu, Ca.: Malibu Publishing Co., 1989.

Juhan, Deanne, *Job's Body,*Barrytown, NY: Station Hill Press, 1987.

Koch, Liz, *Core Awareness,* North Atlantic Books, Berkeley, California, 2012.

Lipton, Bruce H., *The Biology of Belief:* New York, Hay House, Inc.,2005

Milne, Hugh, *The Heart of Listening,* Berkeley, Ca.: North Atlantic Books, 1995.

Olsen, Andrea, *Body Stories: A guide to Experiential Anatomy,* Barrytown, NY: Station Hill Press, 1991.

Oschman, James, *Energy Medicine,* New York: Butterworth Heinemann, 2000

Pollack, Gerald H, *The Fourth Phase of Water,* Ebner and Sons Pub. Seattle, Wash., 2013.

Pollack, Gerald H. *Cells, Gels, and the Engines of Life,* Ebner and Sons Pub. Seattle, Wash. 2001.

Raheem, Aminah, *Soul Return, Integrating Body, Psyche and Spirit,* California, Asia Publishing, 1991.

Ridley, Charles, *Stillness: Biodynamic Cranial Practice and The Evolution of Consciousness,* Berkeley, Ca.: North Atlantic Books, 2006

Rolf, Ida, *Rolfing*

Schleip, Findley, Chaitow, Hujing, *Fascia, The Tensional Network of the Human Body,* Churchill Livingstone, 2012, London.

Schultz, R and Feitis, Rosemary: *The Endless Web,* Berkeley, Ca. North Atlantic Books, l996.

Sills, Franklin, *Craniosacral Biodynamics, Vol. 1&2,* Berkeley, Ca., North Atlantic Books, 2001.

Smith, Fritz, *Inner Bridges,* Atlanta, Ga., Humanics New Age, 1986.

Stone, R. *Polarity Therapy,* Sebastopol, Ca.: CRCS Publications, 1986.

Sutherland, W. *Teachings in the Science of Osteopathy,* Ed, Anne L. Wales, Forth Worth, Tx: Sutherland Cranial Teaching Foundation, 1990.

Upledger, John, *Craniosacral Therapy,* Seattle, Wash.: Eastland Press, 1983.

WEBSITES

Robert Scheip, www.somatic.de www.fascialfitnesstoday.com

J.C. Gimberteau, www.guimberteau-jc-md.com/en

Integral Anatomy, Gill Hedley, www.integralanatomy.com

Dr. Stephen Levin, www.biotensegrity.com

Fascial Conduction, www.fascialconduction.com

GLOSSARY

actin filaments—Strands of collagen molecules containing the globular protein actin, which functions as a contractive mechanism.

awareness—The ability of microtubules and the microfibril/organized water matrix to sense the functioning, moving, relating organism.

adaptability—The ability to respond to external and internal inputs in a quick and integrated way.

balanced reciprocal tension—The ability of a matrix to maintain a balance between the push and pull, compressive and tensile forces, and suspension and coherence.

biotensegrity—The reciprocal tension in living organisms that comes from the balance of tensile and compressive forces, with fascia and muscles being the tensile forces and bones being the compressive forces.

bioelectric field—A field of coherent energy in a living organism that is electrically charged and can conduct a wave current through it.

bioelectric matrix—A charged matrix in a living organism that can conduct wave currents through it.

bound water—Organized water in a container, where protons cluster in the middle of the container and electrons create a zone on either side of them, creating a charged, conductive medium.

coherence—The ability to keep different parts of a system interconnected while each part maintains its own identity. In a living system, coherence is the capacity to store incoming energy in a coherent form, closing the energy loop (so the energy does not drain away to entropy) into a regenerating life cycle.

collagen—A type of protein found in mammals that creates the fiber structure for the connective tissue in the body. There are 14 known types of collagen that form in triplets, first as a molecule of tropocollagen, then into three spiraling fibers as fibrils and collagen fibers.

collagen fibers—Fibers made of microfibrils, which are made of tropocollagen strands that spiral together in threes. They loosely bind water between them, creating a conductive pathway. The organized water/microfibril unit is the internal matrix of the fascia.

conductive field—A confluence of energy that creates a pathway for currents of energy, particles and wave patterns to move.

connective tissue—A type of animal tissue created out of mesodermic stem cells that supports, connects and separates other tissues in the body. All connective tissue consists of fibers, ground substance and cells.

consciousness—The ability of an organism to be aware of itself in relationship to its surroundings and the whole. Sentience, awareness, interconnectedness and memory define consciousness's scope in the body and the mind.

cytoskeleton—The internal matrix of the cell, made up of microfilaments, filaments and microtubules. It is like the internal matrix of the fascia in that it structures, supports, organizes and moves the cell.

density—The amount of mass in a substance per unit of space. The compactness of substance in space.

ectoderm—The outer layer of stem cells in the embryo, which forms the central and peripheral nervous system, epidermis and sense organs.

embodiment—The ability to be aware of the sensations of the body and to experience the world from the body. To be "embodied" means to perceive from the wholeness of your physical being.

embryo—The early stage of development of a human from fertilization of the egg into a multicellular diploid eukaryote, until the third month of pregnancy when it is called a fetus.

endoderm—The inner layer of stem cells during development of the embryo. It forms the inner linings of digestive, respiratory, and auditory tubes; the linings of the thyroid and thymus glands; and the urinary bladder.

energy field—Energy organized around a function, intention or fulcrum, which creates a semipermeable invisible membrane, attracting to it all that enhances its function and repelling all that deconstructs it.

enliven—To energize, stimulate, or give life and spirit to. In the fascial matrix, to enliven means to activate the microfibrils/organized water matrix to shift and change, reconnecting with the whole.

fascia—The interconnected webbing throughout the body that consists of a microfibril/organized water matrix, ground substance and various types of cells. It touches all of the tissues in the body and conducts wave patterns through its matrix.

fascial matrix—The part of fascia that consists of triple helix-spiraled microfibrils with bound (organized) water between the fibrils. This matrix is able to shift and change its microfibril connections in response to pressure and input. This matrix is able to conduct protons, photons and the signature wave motions of the person throughout it completely and immediately.

felt sense—Another sensing mechanism of the body when in awareness. It is a body experience or inner knowledge that hasn't been interpreted by the cognitive brain. The term was first used by psychotherapist Eugene Gendlin in his work called Focusing.

fibroblasts—Large, flat, spindle-shaped cells found in all connective tissue and that secrete and synthesize different types of collagen into the extracellular matrix. Fibroblasts also are important in tissue repair and have an ability to know their location in the organism.

fractal—A continuous pattern that repeats itself in a self-similar way throughout different sizes and scales. Fractals are created in nature through repeating a pattern from macro- to micro-levels.

ground substance—The gel-like fluid that consists of glycosoaminoglycans (GAGs) that surround cells and the matrix in the fascia and have a strong ability to draw water to them.

glide—The ability to move smoothly, effortlessly and evenly without friction or resistance.

hologram—An image, usually made from a laser, that appears three-dimensional and that, when divided even to the tiniest fragment, will continue to show the whole image.

hyaluronic acid – A glycosoaminoglycan found in the ground substance of the fascia that helps with smoothness and glide between the fascia and other tissues. When in excess, it can cause tissues and fascia to bind together.

icosahedron—One of the Platonic solids structures found in nature, comprised of 20 equilateral triangles, where five meet together at 12 points in the structure.

inertial pattern—A part of a matrix isolated from the whole matrix pattern, separating it from the conduction and integral relationship functions of the fascial matrix. Inertial patterns can form their own conductive and relationship pattern.

interstitial fluids—Fluids surrounding cells in an organism, found in the interstitial spaces. They can include extracellular fluid, plasma and transcellular fluid.

ions—Charged atoms or molecules where the number of protons to electrons is unequal. More electrons than protons create a negative ion. More protons than electrons create a positive ion.

lemniscate—A figure eight shape; a curve or infinity symbol. It is a fractal movement pattern found in the body around the midline and within the fascial matrix.

liquid crystalline matrix—The global network of microfibrils and bound water in the fascia that appears crystalline in its coherent ability to conduct information and create memory, while continually shifting and changing connections.

matrix—An interconnected pattern of lines and spaces creating a webbing for other things to form and function within.

mesodermic field—The embryological resonance that invokes the qualities of the primitive streak or first wave of life, the midline of the body and the connection of the three types of stem cells.

mesoderm—The middle layer formed by the primitive streak in the embryo; forming the connective tissue in the body.

microfibrils—Collagen fibers that are spiraled together in threes with organized water (bind water) inside and between them in the fascial matrix.

microfibril/organized water matrix—The matrix within the fascia that creates the balanced reciprocal tension, buoyancy and conductive pathway for the body. It is also called the liquid crystalline matrix.

microtubules—The tubulin protein structures in eukaryotic cells that maintain the shape of the cell, help in cell division, and make movement of the cell possible. Its hollow structure gives it the ability to organize water within it, creating a conductive pathway. They are part of the cytoskeleton of the cell.

microfilaments—Protein fibers that make up the cytoskeleton of cells. They help in shape, cell division and movement of organelles in the cell, as well as movement of the cell. The protein in them varies according to their function.

mobility—The ability of tissue to move and adapt in diverse, quick, responsive ways.

morphogenetic field—A field that organizes around a signal, function or idea, creating a pattern and a memory of its view.

motility—The ability of tissue to move energy out from a center, to move a substance through a pathway, or to respond to an input by moving it forward.

mutability—The ability to shift and change with input. In the fascial matrix, mutability is the ability to shift the microfibril connections while maintaining an integrated, whole conductive pathway.

organized water—Water that has been organized by a tubular container with negative charges on the outside and positive charges in the inside. Also called "structured water."

piezoelectric—The state of a substance (usually crystalline) that becomes electrically charged when a force or pressure is applied to it.

potency—The body's reserve and potential of free flowing energy that can be utilized when the normal functioning of the body is insufficient to respond to input.

protein polymers—Large molecules made up of repeating protein subunits.

In the fascial matrix, the microfibrils are made of tropocollagen subunits that arrange in repeating triads of type 1 collagen protein.

primitive streak—The vibration that moves through the bilaminal disc in the embryo at day 14, creating the mesodermic stem cell layer.

quantum field—The attractions and interaction between at least two systems (particles) where there is a constant relationship and exchange of information.

quantum physics—A theory in physics based on the concept that energy is made of tiny particles (for example, photons make up radiant energy) that can transfer and transform energy, affecting the atomic or molecular state.

resonance – A state when individual vibrations attune to each other, shifting both vibrations to become similar and resonant.

responsive shifting fulcrums – Points of balanced reciprocal tension in the matrix created in response to pressure, movement or wave pattern inputs.

signature wave—The unique, individual changing wave pattern that pulsates through the microfibril/organized water matrix in the fascia.

space-time continuum—The linear progression of time at a certain position in space. It is the present moment that we experience in life.

stem cell—An unspecialized cell that differentiates into a functional, specialized cell in the body through pressure and movement.

suspension—The ability of a substance to mix particles or molecules within it without dissolving or changing those particles.

tensegrity—A portmanteau of the words tension + integrity; the state of a structure that is composed of isolated, compressed parts inside a webbing of continuous tension.

vacuole—A small cavity or space in tissues or in an organism containing fluid.

vitality—The aliveness of an organism that creates tonus and readiness in its tissues to respond to the demands of the internal and external environments.

wave pattern—A disturbance or variance that transfers energy progressively from one point to another, where the movement has a repeating rise and fall pattern.

INDEX

A

Adaptability dimension, 33
Aging, liquid crystalline matrix and,
    147–148
Alignment, shifting fulcrums and, 208

B

Balance, inherent, 202
Balanced reciprocal tension
    balancing reciprocal tensions, 226
    buoyancy or compression, 109–110
    complexity of microfibril/organized
        water matrix, 135–136
    creation of, 108, 138–139
    dynamic nature of, 206
    effects of, 138
    finding directions of tension in body,
        133
    finding your, 109
    gliding around layers of tension, 135
    hands-on unwinding, with partner, 141
    impairment of, 139–140
    layers of balanced tension, 134
    midline as neutral, 134
    overview of, 130–131
    polarity, compression and
        multidimensional tension, 132
    pulling up slack to let tissue unwind,
        139
    touch's effect on, 140–141

Barrett, Sondra, 161, 163, 166, 203
Bilateral injury problem case, 264–266
Bioelectric field, characteristics of, 25
Biotensegrity
    biotensegrity pattern, 17
    creation of term, 163
    finding your, 165
    from tensegrity to, 161–164
Body consciousness, 174
Brain consciousness, 173–174
Brain wave pattern, 79–80
Breath, feeling pulsations of life, 221
Buoyancy, balanced reciprocal tension,
    109–110

C

Case studies
    bilateral injury problems, 264–266
    disconnected conductivity and effects of
        hip replacement, 85
    dry eye and gliding conjunctiva, 69–70
    embodiment, finding signature wave,
        263–264
    excess fluid, tightening boundaries,
        260–261
    full-body density, changing perceptions,
        261–263
    hyperextension and compression in
        matrix, 114–115
    integrating left and right, balancing
        coherent boundary, 128–129

intrinsic and extrinsic matrix disconnect, 100–101
shifting density into fluidity through movement, 50–52
Cells
cell matrix fibers, 169
cell recognition, 203
memory of stem cell possibility, 184–185
suspension within, 106–107
tensegrity in, 166
Chaos theory, fractal design and, 158
Circular pulsation and wave motion, 224
Coherence
balanced reciprocal tension, 108, 256
cohesion vs., 122
conductivity and, 76–77
creation in
fascial field, 118–119
fascial structure, 117–118
crystal memory and, 120–121
defined, 117
effects of, 124
feeling
change in coherence around inertial patterns, 125
pull of, 126
field of relationship, 120
fractal design and, 157–158, 159
inertial patterns and, 124
integrating left and right, balancing coherent boundary, 128–129
in microfibrils/organized water matrix, 119
overview of, 116–117
stability vs. mutability, 122–123
suspension and, 108
touching coherence, with partner, 127
touch's effect on, 125–126
Coherent awareness, 177–178
experiencing, through matrix, 179
Cohesion, coherence vs., 122
Collagen fibers
characteristics of, 16
in fascia, 170–171
formation from fibroblasts, 16
fractal collagen fibers to microfibrils,

152
as internal structure of fascia, 16
Compartmentalization
interrelationship vs. isolation, 94–95
process of, 93
Compression
areas of compression, overstretch or immobility, 256–257
balanced reciprocal tension, 109–110
compress and glide, 237
finding, 226–227
hyperextension and compression in matrix, 114–115
moving compressive and tensile forces, 248–250
opening compressive holding patterns, 227–228
Conductive field
characteristics of, 25
creating slide and glide in, 58
creation of, 74–75
feeling, 28
Conductivity
coherence vs. dispersion, 76–77
conduction vs. disconnect, 75–76
creating in fascia, 73–74
creating in field, 74–75
disconnects, and effects of hip replacement, 85
effects of, 82
feeling in body, 72
inertial patterns in, 83, 85
levels of, 258–259
mesodermic relationships in, 77–78
overview of, 71–72
patterns of, 79–80
touch's effect on, 83–84
Conjunctiva, dry eyes and gliding, 69–70
Connective tissue
structure of, 23–24
types of, 24
Conscious awareness, 177
Consciousness
body consciousness, 174
brain consciousness, 173–174
conscious awareness, 177
matrix consciousness, 174–176

survival and, 176–177
Cranial tide, 221
Crystalline biolectric matrix, 92–93
Crystal memory
    characteristics of, 120–121
    liquid crystalline matrix and, 143
    moving within, 122
Cytoskeleton, of cell, suspension and,
    106–107

D

Density, 35–53
    characteristics of, 36
    compared to fluidity, 43
    creating
        in fascia, 37–39
        in field, 39–40
    effects of, 44
    finding layers of, 37
    full-body density, changing perceptions
        case, 261–263
    gel/sol, 40–41
    inertial pattern, 39, 44–46
    massage techniques, 252–253
    palpation of, 44
    piezoelectric effect, 49
    resistance vs. resilience, 41–42
    shifting, into fluidity through
        movement, 50–52
    thickness vs. sponginess, 42–43
    touch's effect on, 48–49
Direct massage techniques, 250–251
Dispersion, conductivity and, 77
Dry eye, and gliding conjunctiva, 69–70
Dural tube, 12
Dura mater, 12

E

Earth tide, 222
Ectoderm, 22
    midline, 191
Electromagnetic field, signature wave and,
    62–63
Embryo
    fascia developing from, 22–23
    layering of fascia, 90–91

primitive streak in, 22–23
Embryonic field potential, 187
Endoderm, 22
    midline, 192
Energy field
    bioelectric field, 25
    bridge between structure and field, 31
    of conductive field, 25
    defined, 25
    mesodermic field, 26
    morphogenetic field, 26
Entangle rhythms, 204
Enteroception, 33
Explorations
    balancing reciprocal tension, with
        partners, 142
    complexifying our microfibril
        connections, 137
    connecting
        internal and external matrix, 123
        liquid crystalline matrix from cell to
            fascia to world, 172
    engaging
        inherent health, 202
        self-regulating system, 200
    experiencing coherent awareness
        through matrix, 179
    feeling
        change in coherence around inertial
            patterns, 125
        coherence in matrix, 118
        conductive field, 28
        conductivity in body, 72
        conductivity in hands, 82
        impaired reciprocal tension,
            139–140
        piezoelectric effect, 49
        pull of coherence, 126
        slide and glide in hands, 64
    fields of resonance and layers of wave in
        body, 30
    finding
        conductivity inertial patterns on
            partner, 85
        directions of tension in body, 133
        fascial matrix, 19
        fulcrum level of stillness, 207

inertial patterns of density, 46
layers of density, 37
layers within field, 91
mesodermic connections, 78
microfibril/organized water matrix
in our hands, 236
mutable mesodermic layers, 189
our fractal design, 153
stem cell potency, 186
suspension in body, 107
your balanced reciprocal tension,
109
your biotensegrity, 165
your heart coherence, 198
your mesodermic midline, 193
your patterns of conductivity, 81
your signature wave, 63
your slide and glide, 55
finding your SA node, 197
fluid movement, 47
fractal design and coherence, 159
gliding
around layers of tension, 135
your inertial patterns, 65–66
hands-on unwinding, with partner, 141
lubricating surface of fascia, 57
moving
with coherence field, 119
within crystal memory, 122
functional matrix, 21
lemniscate around midline, 157
from shifting matrix to shifting
fulcrum, 209
palpation of density, 44
pulling up slack to let tissue unwind,
139
reconnecting layers of fascia, 94
sensing our entangled signature wave,
205
shifting from muscle movement to
fascial movement, 14–15
suspending
your internal patterns, 112
your psoas, 111
touching
coherence, with partner, 127
and dancing with liquid crystalline

matrix, 149
layers of matrix, 98–99
suspension in fascia, 113
tuning your microfibril dance, 146
using hands to slide and glide partner's
matrix, 69
variance of glide, motility and mobility, 67
Exteroception, 33

F

Falx celebri, 12
Falx cerebelli, 12
Fascia
coherence creation in, 117–118
collagen fibers, 16, 170–171
conductivity creation in, 73–74
defined, 11–12
density creation in, 37–39
development of, in embryo, 22–23
fibroblast, 16
function of, 20
gliding, 214–217
gliding superficial fascia, 225
ground substance, 15–16
internal structure, 15–16
layering creation, 88–90
layers overview, 11–12
lubricating, 57
overview of qualities, 32–34
reconnecting layers of fascia, 94
slide and glide creation in, 55–56
spiraling and moving fascia, 219–220
suspension creation in, 103–104
tensegrity in, 166
Fascial Conduction, 233–259
ability to resonate signature wave to
external matrix, 259
areas of compression, overstretch or
immobility, 256–257
balancing reciprocal tensions of
compressive/tensile forces, 248–
250, 256–259
case studies of, 260–266
coherence/suspension, 256
contacting the field, 238–240
contacting the structure, 236–238

creating impulse, 240–241
finding microfibril/organized water
    matrix in our hands, 236
inertial patterns, 257–258
levels of conductivity, 258–259
making contact: matrix to matrix, 235–
    236, 243–244
massage techniques applied to, 250–256
moving compressive and tensile forces,
    248–250
overview of, 233–235
reestablishing midline fulcrum, 247–
    248
slide and glide (impulse and stream),
    244–246
streaming, 241–242
what to expect as client, 242–243
Fascial field
bridge between structure and field, 31
coherence creation in, 118–119
defined, 26
key components of, 27
layering creation in, 90
suspension creation in, 104–105
Fascial function, 25
Fascial matrix
contacting the structure, 236–238
finding your, 19
making contact: matrix to matrix, 235–
    236, 243–244
moving, 48
Fascial movement, shifting to, from muscle
    movement, 14–15, 213
Feeling the pulsations of life: breath, 221
Feitis, R., 12, 20, 23
Fiber connections
cell matrix fibers, 169
fascial matrix fibers, 170–171
microtubules and, 169–170
Fibroblast
characteristics of, 16
as internal structure of collagen fiber, 16
Field. *See also* Energy field
complexity of patterns in, 204
contacting, 238–240
defined, 25
density creation in, 39–40

slide and glide creation in, 58
Field of relationship, 120
Figure 8
around spine and joints, 218–219
in Fascial Conduction, 237
reestablishing midline fulcrum, 247–
    248
Floating compression, 167–168
Fluidity
compared to density, 43
shifting density into, through
    movement, 50–52
Fluid movement, 47
Formless awareness, 178
Fractal design
chaos theory and, 158
coherence and, 157–158, 159
complexity of, 153–154
defined, 150–152
finding our, 153
fractal collagen fibers to microfibrils,
    152
lemniscate, 156–157
linear vs. multidirectional impulse,
    154–156
Fulcrums
alignment and, 208
defined, 206
finding fulcrum level of stillness, 207
moving from shifting matrix to shifting
    fulcrum, 209
responsive shifting fulcrums, 207–208
Fuller, Buckminster, 161–162
Functional matrix, moving, 21

G

Gel/sol, 40–41
    massage techniques and, 252–253
Gintis, Bonnie, 61, 187, 189, 201, 208
Glide. *See* Slide and glide
Gravity, changing relationship to, 217
Ground substance
characteristics of, 15–16
gel/sol, 40–41
as internal structure of fascia, 15–16
Guimberteau, Jean-Claude, 3, 144, 164, 176

H

Hands-on practice. *See* Fascial Conduction
Heartbeat, 221
Heart coherence
    characteristics of, 195–196
    finding your, 198
Heart rate wave pattern, 79–80
Heart resonance, 195
Hip replacement, disconnected conductivity
    effects on, 85
Ho, Mae-Wan, 17, 121, 158, 173, 204
Horizontal diaphragms, 12
Hyaluronic acid, creating slide and glide in
    fascia, 55–57
Hyperextension in matrix, 114–115

I

Immobility, areas of, 256–257
Impulse
    creating, 240–241
    initiating, 223
    slide and glide, 244–246
Indirect massage techniques, 250–251
Inertial patterns, 39
    coherence and, 124
    in conductivity, 83, 85
    density in, 44–46
    Fascial Conduction and, 257–258
    feeling change in coherence around
        inertial patterns, 125
    finding, 46, 229
    finding through layers, 98
    gliding through, 229–230
    gliding your, 66
    layering and, 97
    self-practice for, 229
    slide and glide in, 66
    streaming through, 230
Ingber, Donald, 162–163
Inherent health, 201, 202
Internal matrix
    bridge between structure and field, 31
    concepts in, moving, 182–183
    enlivening, 180
    importance of, 4
    repairing, 5–6
    as whole organism, 3–4
Internal patterns, in suspension, 111–112
Interrelationship, isolation vs., 94–95
Isolation, interrelationship vs, 94–95

J

Joints, figure 8 around spine and joints,
    218–219

L

Layering
    of balanced tension, 134
    compartmentalization, 93
    creation in fascial field, 90
    creation in fascial structure, 88–90
    effects of, 96
    engaging deeper layers, 226
    engaging layers while gliding and
        streaming, 224
    fascial layers as webbing, 91–92
    finding deeper layers, 230
    finding layers within field, 91
    internal patterns and, 97, 98
    interrelationship vs. isolation, 94–95
    intrinsic and extrinsic matrix disconnect
        case, 100–101
    massage techniques, 255–256
    microfibril/organized water layers as
        crystalline biolectric matrix, 92–93
    mobility, motility and mutability, 95
    overview of, 87–88
    reconnecting layers of fascia, 94
    touch's effect on, 98–99
Lemniscate
    characteristics of, 156–157
    moving around your midline, 157
    reestablishing midline fulcrum, 247–
        248
Levin, Stephen M., 160–161, 163–164
Linear impulse, fractal design and, 154–156
Lipton, Bruce, 120
Liquid crystalline matrix, 45
    aging and, 147–148
    concepts to remember when engaging,
        212

connecting liquid crystalline matrix
from cell to fascia to world, 172
crystal memory and, 143
defined, 143
mutability and stability, 146–147
overview of, 143
as seat of consciousness, 171
touch's effect on, 148–149
watching microfibrils move and change,
144–145
Longitudinal tide, Earth tide, 222
Lubrication
dry eye and gliding conjunctiva, 69–70
of fascia with hyaluronic acid, 57

M

Massage techniques applied to Fascial
Conduction, 250–256
direct and indirect methods, 250–252
gel/sol, 252–253
quality of density, 252–253
quality of glide, 254–255
quality of layering, 255–256
techniques for working structure/field,
252
Matrix consciousness
activity and, 175–176
characteristics of, 174–175
through coherent matrix, 175
Mechanotransduction, 162–163
Mesenchyme, 187–188
Mesoderm, 22
finding mutable mesodermic layers, 189
mesodermic relationships in
conductivity, 77–78
midline, 191
Mesodermic field
characteristics of, 26
memory, 188
Mesodermic field memory, 188
Mesoderm midline
characteristics of, 191, 192
finding your, 193
uses of, 193–194
Microfibrils
biotensegrity pattern, 17

formation of, 16
fractal collagen fibers to microfibrils, 152
watching, move and change, 144–145
Microfibrils/organized water matrix
balanced reciprocal tension, 108
characteristics of, 17–18
coherence in, 119
complexity of, and balanced reciprocal
tension, 135–136
conductivity creation and, 73–74
finding microfibril/organized water
matrix in our hands, 236
function of, 22
layers as crystalline biolectric matrix,
92–93
suspension creation and, 104–105
Microtubules, fiber connection and,
169–170
Midline
ectoderm, 191
endoderm, 192
gliding, 231–232
as main fulcrum for body, 207
mesoderm, 191, 192–194
as neutral and balanced reciprocal
tension, 134
stillness and, 231
streaming from, 232
Midline fulcrum, reestablishing, 247–248
Midline tide, 222
Mobility
finding your, 96
healthy, defined, 61
layering and, 95
slide and glide, 61–62, 67
Morphogenetic field, 26
Motility
characteristics of, 61–62
finding your, 96
layering and, 95
slide and glide, 61–62, 67
Multidimensional tension, balanced
reciprocal tension and, 132
Multidirectional impulse, fractal design and,
154–156
Muscle movement, shifting to fascial
movement from, 14–15, 213

Mutability
  coherence and, 122–123
  finding your, 96
  layering and, 95
  liquid crystalline matrix, 146–147
Myofascia, defined, 11

O

Organized water matrix. *See* Microfibrils/
  organized water matrix
Overstretch, areas of, 256–257

P

Patterns, unwinding, 230
Pelvic diaphragm, 12
Piezoelectric effect
  characteristics of, 49
  feeling, 49
Polarity, balanced reciprocal tension and, 132
Potency dimension, 32
Primitive streak
  characteristics of, 22–23, 190
  layering and, 90
Proprioception, 33
Proton pump, 17, 62–63

R

Recalibration and renewal, 231
Reciprocal tension. *See also* Balanced
  reciprocal tension
  balancing, 248–250
Resilience, density and, 41–42
Resistance, density and, 41–42
Resonance
  characteristics of, 29
  defined, 24–25, 29
  fields of, 30
  from glide to resonance, 220
Resources in body, for moving internal
  matrix, 182–183
Respiratory diaphragm, 12
Responsive shifting fulcrums, 207–208
  alignment and, 208
  moving from shifting matrix to, 209
Retinacular cutis, 89

Ridley, Charles, 144, 152, 154, 158, 192,
  196, 201

S

Schultz, R., 12, 20, 23
Self-practice, 210–233
  balancing reciprocal tensions, 226
  basic sequence, 211, 213
  benefits of, 210–211
  changing relationship to gravity, 217
  circular pulsation and wave motion, 224
  concepts to engage liquid crystalline
    matrix, 212
  cranial tide, 221
  engaging
    deeper layers, 226
    layers while gliding and streaming,
      224
  feeling the pulsations of life: breath, 220
  figure 8 around spine and joints,
    218–219
  finding
    compression and tensile forces,
      226–227
    deeper layers, 230
    inertial patterns, 229
  from glide to resonance, 220
  gliding
    the fascia, 214–217
    the midline, 231–232
    superficial fascia, 225
    through inertial patterns, 229–230
  heartbeat, 221
  inertial patterns, 229
  initiating impulse and streaming, 223
  longitudinal tide, Earth tide, 222
  midline and stillness, 231
  midline tide, 222
  opening compressive holding patterns,
    227–228
  recalibration and renewal, 231
  spiraling and moving fascia, 219–220
  streaming
    from midline, 232
    through inertial patterns, 230
  unwinding patterns, 230

warm up: muscle movement to fascial
    movement, 213
Self-recognition
    cell recognition, 203
    complexity of patterns in field, 204
    entangle rhythms, 204
    signature wave and, 205
Self-regulating system
    benefits of, 199–200
    engaging, 200
Self-sustaining system, 199–200
Shoulder diaphragm, 12
Signature wave
    ability to resonate signature wave to
        external matrix, 259
    characteristics of, 9–10
    electromagnetic field and, 62–63
    embodiment, finding signature wave
        case, 263–264
    entangled, 205
    finding your, 63
    proton pump and, 17, 62–63
    self-recognition and, 205
Sinoatrial node
    characteristics of, 196
    finding your, 197
Sleeve, layering of fascial structure, 88–89
Slickness, slide and glide, 60–61
Slide and glide
    compress and glide, 237
    creating
        in fascia, 55–56
        in field, 58
    dry eye and gliding conjunctiva, 69–70
    effects of, 64
    engaging layers while gliding and
        streaming, 224
    in Fascial Conduction, 237, 244–246
    feeling in hands, 64
    finding your, 55
    from glide to resonance, 220
    gliding
        around layers of tension, 135
        the fascia, 214–217
        the midline, 231–232
        superficial fascia, 225
        tensile and compressive forces, 249

through inertial patterns, 229–230
hyaluronic acid and, 55–57
impulse and stream, 244–246
inertial patterns, 65–66
massage techniques for areas with
    limited, 254–255
mobility vs. motility, 61–62, 67
overview of, 53–54
signature wave and electromagnetic
    field, 62–63
stickiness vs. slickness, 60–61
touch's effect on, 68
variations of, 59–60
Snelson, Kenneth, 167–168
Sol, 40–41
Spine, figure 8 around spine and joints,
    218–219
Sponginess, density and, 42–43
Starfish streaming, 223
Stem cells
    characteristics of, 184
    development of, 185
    finding stem cell potency, 186
    mesenchyme, 187–188
Stickiness, slide and glide, 60–61
Streaming
    defined, 241
    engaging layers while gliding and
        streaming, 224
    in Fascial Conduction, 241–242
    initiating, 223
    from midline, 232
    slide and glide, 244–246
    through inertial patterns, 230
Superficial fascia, gliding, 225
Suspension
    balanced reciprocal tension, 108
    in body, 105
    buoyancy or compression, 109–110
    within cells, 106–107
    coherence and, 108
    components of, 103
    creation in fascial field, 104–105
    creation in fascial structure, 103–104
    defined, 103
    effects of, 110
    in facial structure, 105

finding in body, 107
hyperextension and compression in
     matrix, 114–115
internal patterns in, 111–112
touching suspension in fascia, 113
touch's effect on, 112–113

Wave motion, circular pulsation and, 224
Webbing
     fascial layers as, 91–92
     suspension in body and, 105
Western medicine, concepts of, 182–183

T

Tensegrity
     in cells, 166
     defined, 160
     in fascia, 166
     floating compression, 167–168
     from, to biotensegrity, 161–164
     qualities of tensegrity structures in body,
          165
Tensile forces
     finding, 226–227
     moving, 248–250
     opening compressive holding patterns,
          227–228
Tentorium cerebelli, 12
Thickness, density and, 42–43
Touch, effect of
     balanced reciprocal tension, 140–141
     coherence, 125–126
     conductivity, 83–84
     density, 48–49
     layering, 98–99
     on liquid crystalline matrix, 148–149
     slide and glide, 68
     suspension, 112–113
Tropocollagen molecules, 16

V

Visceral fascia, 12
Vitality
     inherent, 202
     vitality dimension, 33

W

Wave
     entangle rhythms, 204
     layers of, in body, 30
     signature wave, 9–10

ABOUT THE AUTHOR
LIBBY OUTLAW, LMBT, SOMATIC EDUCATOR

I feel privileged and honored to have observed and explored the internal matrices of hundreds of people during my hands-on career as a bodywork practitioner, and I have come to respect deeply the internal matrix's role in our overall health and consciousness.

After finishing college with a BA in Economics and International Studies at American University in 1972, I changed directions and began my lifetime study and career as a therapeutic massage and bodywork practitioner. After studying a system that included Rolfing, Gestalt Therapy and Polarity Therapy, I taught and practiced bodywork while traveling with my first husband throughout the Southeastern United States. I continued my studies by exploring Chinese Medicine, traveling to China to study TCM and TuiNa. I also trained in many neuromuscular and fascial techniques, such as Neuromuscular Therapy, Structural Bodywork, the Bowen Method, Myofascial Release and Cranial Sacral Therapy. For 12 years I was a faculty member at the Carolina School of Massage Therapy, teaching Deep Muscle Massage, Acupressure and Case Studies. I contributed to the development of the curriculum at the school, creating a Deep Muscle Handbook and serving as Education Director.

During my 40 years of working with hundreds of clients, I have learned a great deal about the diversity, adaptability and habitual nature of the body. For years I have worked with resistance in the soft tissue, blocks in the meridian system, and imbalances in the cranial system.

Over the years, exploring these many fields, I always sensed the presence of a connector, an integrator that I was not touching in my work. Then, around eighteen years ago, I began to investigate the fascial matrix as this possible connector, and I was amazed by the scientific research of Mae-Wan Ho and the videos of Dr. Guimbierteau. With this work as a starting point, I began in earners to develop new methods to address the body's soft tissue as a bio-electric matrix of relationship. This evolved into the work of Fascial Conduction (see website www.fascialconduction.com). From the vast array of human matrix configurations, I have learned to decipher the enlivened matrix from the inertial patterns. This has led me to develop an experiential exploration of this matrix and to create ways to enhance its complexity and adaptability.

I have been engaged in a long-term Authentic Movement and Continuum Movement practice in the Chapel Hill area. My exploration in these free, diverse movement expressions and my own internal and movement practices have created in me a more complex, diverse moving body. All of this has informed the directions given in this book for the self-practice of moving the internal matrix.

Because of my research, my life is rich in many other ways, all that inform my conductive field, from working in the rich soils at Maple Spring Gardens, an organic farm that I own with my husband in Cedar Grove, North Carolina , to tending my sacred garden, to teaching and writing and moving and creating. Thus this book is a synthesis of my professional and embodied life.

Made in the USA
San Bernardino, CA
17 November 2016